What if successful people define themselves as verbs, not as nouns? As doers, not as objects? Amanda Brouwer skillfully illuminates how to use this technique to become a healthier eater, as well as an effective "doer" more generally.

—Kennon M. Sheldon, Curators' Distinguished Professor of Psychological Sciences, University of Missouri

Motivation for Sustaining Health Behavior Change

With a balance of theory, research, and applications, *Motivation for Sustaining Health Behavior Change: The Self-as-Doer Identity* introduces the self-as-doer identity as an accessible motivational identity and discusses how it can be incorporated into health behavior change efforts. The book introduces the self-as-doer theory and presents research and recommendations for how the self-as-doer can be used in both clinical and non-clinical populations to promote health behavior change and maintenance. The book will be of interest to researchers, students, and professionals interested in health promotion.

Amanda M. Brouwer is Associate Professor of Psychology at Winona State University, USA. She teaches social, health, and quantitative statistics to undergraduates and studies how psychosocial concepts such as identity and self-efficacy influence health behavior enactment. She has published in journals such as *Self and Identity*, *Qualitative Health Research*, *The Diabetes Educator*, *Archives of Sexual Behavior*, and *Chronic Illness*.

Motivation for Sustaining Health Behavior Change

The Self-as-Doer Identity

Amanda M. Brouwer

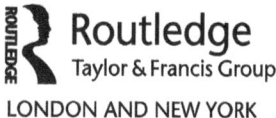

Routledge
Taylor & Francis Group

LONDON AND NEW YORK

First published 2018 by Routledge

2 Park Square, Milton Park, Abingdon, Oxfordshire OX14 4RN

52 Vanderbilt Avenue, New York, NY 10017

Routledge is an imprint of the Taylor & Francis Group, an informa business

First issued in paperback 2019

Library of Congress Cataloging-in-Publication Data
A catalog record for this book has been requested

ISBN: 978-1-138-03635-2 (hbk)
ISBN: 978-0-367-26633-2 (pbk)

Typeset in Times New Roman
by Apex CoVantage, LLC

Contents

Preface   viii
Acknowledgments   x
Contributors   xi

1 **A Primer on Health, Health Behavior Change, and Identity**   1

2 **The Self-as-Doer: An Introduction**   16
   AMANDA M. BROUWER AND LINDA S. HOUSER-MARKO

3 **Creating Self-as-Doer Identities**   27

4 **Self-as-Doer Identity and Health Behavior Change Within Non-Clinical Populations**   42

5 **Self-as-Doer Identity and Health Behavior Change Within Clinical Populations**   58
   AMANDA M. BROUWER AND KATIE E. MOSACK

6 **Recommendations for Using the Self-as-Doer Identity**   73
   AMANDA M. BROUWER AND KATIE E. MOSACK

Index   89

Preface

I was in a health psychology class in college when I first recognized the depth to which psychological and social factors affect health and health behavior change. As I continued to study I became curious about the degree to which these factors might affect motivation for behavior change, especially for individuals living with chronic illnesses like diabetes and heart disease. With lifestyle factors, which prove difficult to maintain over time, as a major player in the growing rates of such illnesses, I began researching psychological and social factors that affect motivation to engage in and maintain health behavior changes. Among many other reasons, I fell in love with researching the self-as-doer because of its ability to connect psychological and social principles with behavior change. Furthermore, the creativity in which individuals develop and identify with being the doer of their various health behaviors (e.g., "chocolate resister," "size 8 jeans wearer," "more vegetable fitter inner," "moving studier") is insightful. It sometimes elicits laughter in the process of developing serious health goals, but the self-as-doer and the process of working toward becoming that doer, are individually meaningful and personalized. This work reminds me that we as individuals in our pursuit of health are more than just our biological make-up. We are also a product of our psychological and social environments. To that end, I am pleased to share how the self-as-doer identity plays a role in that journey.

I am indebted to many who have helped me reach this point. First, I recognize Mandy Krueger and Jennifer Feenstra who helped me through the first project with the self-as-doer and provided meaningful feedback and support for its continued exploration. I am also immensely grateful for Katie Mosack's ongoing mentorship and contributions to the development of my self-as-doer research. I am especially appreciative of her assistance in the process of writing of this book. Her attention to detail and ability to conceptualize and communicate the larger picture are important parts of the advancement of this work. Finally, thank you to Scott, my spouse, for consistent support through this endeavor.

The purpose of this book is to introduce the self-as-doer identity and how it accounts for motivation and health behavior change (Chapter 2 and Chapter 3), to discuss research and application of the self-as-doer to health behavior change in non-clinical (Chapter 4) and clinical populations (Chapter 5), and to propose ways for the self-as-doer to be used in multiple, diverse settings (Chapter 6). This book has been written in such a way as to appeal to diverse audiences interested in health behavior change and maintenance. However, health care professionals and non-scientists may be particularly interested in chapters discussing the usability and applicability of the self-as-doer in various populations (e.g., Chapters 4, 5, and 6). Those working in clinical and research settings might be specifically interested in chapters describing the development and measurement of the self-as-doer identity (Chapter 3), outcomes of an intervention for the self-as-doer identity (e.g., Chapter 4), and recommendations for its use in other research and clinical contexts (Chapter 6).

Acknowledgments

I would like to acknowledge Mandy Krueger and Jennifer Feenstra for introducing me to the self-as-doer construct and supporting me in the first exploration of its utility and use in a population of individuals with diabetes. I would also like to acknowledge Katie Mosack for her invaluable support in the development and dissemination of research on the self-as-doer identity. Additionally, I am immensely grateful for her feedback and editing throughout the process of writing this book. Finally, thank you to my spouse, Scott, for his ongoing support of all that I aspire to do.

Contributors

Linda S. Houser-Marko is a social and personality psychologist who conducts research on the self, personality, motivation, and well-being along the life course. She is currently a researcher for the Johnson O'Connor Research Foundation. She has an undergraduate degree from Gustavus Adolphus College in Minnesota and a Ph.D. from the University of Missouri, Columbia.

Katie E. Mosack studies topics related to health behavior change and medical self-management among people living with HIV, diabetes, hypertension, and other chronic health conditions. She also studies health care experiences among marginalized populations and has published over 30 journal articles in journals such as *Self and Identity*, *Qualitative Health Research*, *Women's Health Issues*, *Behavioral Medicine*, and *Chronic Illness*.

1 A Primer on Health, Health Behavior Change, and Identity

The World Health Organization defines health as "a complete state of physical, mental and social well-being and not merely the absence of disease or infirmity" (World Health Organization, 1948). Health is a culturally-defined, multidimensional construct. It can be measured as a state of optimal physiological functioning of various body systems (e.g., good blood pressure, strong resting heart rate, absence of pain) as well as in terms of psychological wellness (e.g., mood, depression, stress levels) and engaging in healthy psychological practices (e.g., use good coping skills). One's state of health (e.g., "She is healthy because she engages in physical activity quite regularly") can also be explained as the degree to which individuals engage in health promoting (e.g., eating healthy, being physically active) or health diminishing (e.g., smoking, excessive alcohol consumption) behaviors. From this perspective, health is conceptualized as more than just a biological state; one's well-being is also a result of his or her social and psychological experiences which are then considered important facets of health.

Unfortunately, many people fall short of achieving good health. For instance, only one in five American adults are meeting physical activity recommendations (Center for Disease Control [CDC], 2014) and less than one in ten Americans consume the recommended daily servings of fruit and vegetables (Kimmons, Gillespie, Seymour, Serdula, & Blanck, 2009; Moore & Thompson, 2015). Approximately 3% of the United States population reports experiencing serious psychological distress and are twice as likely to have heart disease or diabetes compared to those who do not experience psychological disease (Weissman, Pratt, Miller, & Parker, 2015). Results from the National Health and Nutrition Examination Survey demonstrate that more than 78% of American adults are overweight or obese (Fryar, Carroll, & Ogden, 2016). Diseases owing to lifestyle factors are becoming more pervasive. The rates of chronic illnesses such as diabetes and cardiovascular disease are growing with approximately 28% of adults having a diagnosis cardiovascular disease and over 1.5 million individuals having diagnosis of diabetes, a number that has tripled since 1980 (CDC, 2015a). Chronic diseases such as heart disease, cancer, and diabetes, which are primarily the result of unhealthy lifestyle behaviors, account for more than 50% of all deaths each year (CDC, 2015b). Others indicate that 40% of premature deaths can be specifically attributed to suboptimal health behaviors (Spruijt-Metz, et al., 2015). That unhealthy lifestyle behaviors are often indicators of the cause of disease diagnosis and progression suggests that health promotion efforts focus on modifying health diminishing behaviors and enhancing health promoting behaviors.

The recommendations for reducing risk of disease and achieving optimal health are to engage in health behaviors such as getting regular physical activity, eating a healthy diet, limiting alcohol consumption, and not using tobacco (CDC, 2015b; Ford, Zhao, Tsai, & Li, 2011; Riekert, Ockene, & Pbert, 2014). Researchers have found that engaging in a combination of these behaviors has potential to decrease mortality risks by 66% (Loef & Walach, 2012). Additionally, Hastert, Ruterbusch, Beresford, Sheppard, and White (2016) found that modifying risk factors (e.g., smoking, diet, physical activity, disease screening rates, etc.) can explain health disparities in cancer mortality rates. The researchers determined that among those with low socioeconomic status, where cancer mortality rates are the highest, the modifiable risk factors could explain as much as 45% of the relationship between socioeconomic status and cancer mortality. Given that the leading causes of death are primarily the result of poor lifestyle behavior choices and that healthy lifestyle choices require self-regulatory behaviors (e.g., choosing to exercise, abstain from tobacco, eat a healthy diet, etc.), optimal health and disease management strategies should then focus on improving lifestyle and health decision-making behaviors.

Healthy lifestyle change is difficult, however. Attrition rates for health behavior change programs are often high and maintenance for successful behavior change is low (Crutzen, Viechtbauer, Spigt, & Kotz, 2015; de Bruin, McCambridge, & Prins, 2015; Dumville, Torgerson, & Hewitt, 2006). Researchers demonstrate that for various forms of health behaviors, individuals are often successful at first, but then struggle to maintain the behavior change. For example, people who enrolled in a healthy eating intervention focused on increasing fruit and vegetable consumption did increase their fruit and vegetable consumption after the intervention, but less than half still maintain those behaviors 6 months after the intervention (Hamel & Robbins, 2013; Lee Olstad et al., 2016). Similar results can be found for weight loss programs. Many successfully lose weight, but then gain the weight back within 3–5 years (Avenell et al., 2004; Dombrowski et al., 2014; Foster et al., 2010). Smoking cessation programs also have poor maintenance outcomes with various interventions (e.g., text messaging, exercise programing, etc.) causing participants to show initial promise for smoking abstinence, but then having high relapse rates at 6- and 12-month follow-ups (Agboola, Mcneill, Coleman, & Leonardi Bee, 2010; Prapavessis et al., 2016; Spohr et al., 2015). Health behavior change is challenging and sustaining changes proves to be even more difficult.

In exploring how to promote health amid the difficulty of making and sustaining changes, it is of value to consider the context in which individuals make health decisions. Again, health is a multifaceted construct influenced by social, psychological, and environmental contexts. Each day, people make choices that can move them more toward poor health (e.g., poor diet, lack of exercise, smoking) or toward more optimal health (e.g., eating well, getting regular physical activity, sleeping well). The factors that influence these decisions are widespread and can vary from day to day, thereby affecting one's ability to make sustaining health behavior change. Individual (idiosyncratic) and contextual barriers to health behavior change exist and reduce the success of making and sustaining needed health behavior change.

Researchers have identified several barriers to engaging in health behaviors including lack of time because of family or occupational responsibilities, difficulty accessing facilities or resources needed to enact the behavior, financial costs, having negative outcome expectancies of engaging in a behavior (e.g., "my back hurts because I worked out"), lack of knowledge to make measurable changes (e.g., "what constitutes a serving of vegetables?"), and the development of certain beliefs and attitudes about health behaviors that then prevent the engagement of that behavior (e.g., "whole grain foods are tasteless and dry," "walking more will only damage my knee further"; Bouma, van Wilgen, & Dijkstra, 2015; Kelly et al., 2016). In proposing ways to overcome barriers to health behavior enactment and given the multidimensional nature of health, it is of value to consider psychological and social factors that can motivate individuals to persist in health behaviors despite the barriers they face. Programs grounded in comprehensive health behavioral models have been more successful in creating and sustaining behavior change than programs not grounded in health behavior change models (Fishbein, 2002; Near & Zimmerman, 2005). Two specific health behavior models merit mention here due to their inclusion of social and psychological variables and how useful they have been in predicting a diverse set health behaviors. They include the Health Belief Model and the Theory of Planned Behavior.

Health Belief Model

The Health Belief Model (HBM) was developed out of a need to better understand and explain why individuals routinely fail to accept and engage in preventative care behaviors like that of early disease screenings

(Rosenstock, 1974). It has since then been extended to describe preventative action, illness behaviors, and sick-role behaviors (Rosenstock, 1990). The model was built to focus on personalized beliefs about disease and disease risk. According to this model, an individual's primary objectives when choosing to engage in health behaviors are to avoid illness and reduce risk of disease (Riekert et al., 2014). More specifically, a health-related behavior will be based on the degree to which one perceives a certain degree of *susceptibility* for contracting a disease or illness and the perceived *severity* of the disease. Before enacting a health behavior, individuals will also consider the *benefits* of engaging in behavior and whether those benefits will outweigh the *barriers* (or costs of) that might prevent the success of reducing susceptibility to or severity of the disease. *Cues to action*, environmental and sociodemographic factors that stimulate the decision-making process (e.g., advice from friends, age, gender, etc.), are also considered important to the process of taking health-related action (Rosenstock, 1990). As Rosenstock (1990) stated,

> it is now believed that individuals will take action to ward off, to screen for, or to control ill-health conditions if they regard themselves as susceptible to the condition, if they believe it to have potentially serious consequences, if they believe that a course of action available to them would be beneficial in reducing either their susceptibility to or severity of the condition, and if they believe that the anticipated barriers to (or costs of) taking the action are outweighed by its benefits.
>
> (pp. 42–43)

The HBM has been used to better understand healthy eating behaviors (Deshpande, Basil, & Basil, 2009; Martinez et al., 2016; Sapp & Weng, 2007), safe sex practices (Asare, Sharma, Bernard, Rojas-Guyler, & Wang, 2013; Wright, Randall, & Hayes, 2012), dental hygiene (Anagnostopoulos, Buchanan, Frousiounioti, Niakas, & Potamianos, 2011; Buglar, White, & Robinson, 2010) and health screening behaviors (Brenner, Ko, Janz, Gupta, & Inadomi, 2015; Lee, Stange, & Ahluwalia, 2015; Sohler, Jerant, & Franks, 2015). In a systematic review of the effectiveness of the HBM in health-related interventions, Jones, Smith, and Llewellyn (2014) determined that barriers and benefits tend to be the strongest predictor of health behaviors whereas there is less support for susceptibility and severity. They also found that the model seemed to best suited to predict primary prevention behaviors (rather than secondary preventative behaviors) and worked most efficiently to predict adherence. Although researchers have found evidence to support the use of the HBM in health behavior interventions, many have argued that the model is limited in that fails to focus on motivational and self-regulatory processes. Nonetheless the HBM has been an integral model in understanding health behavior change and ways to promote health behaviors.

Theory of Reasoned Action and the Theory of Planned Behavior

The Theory of Planned Behavior (TPB) was developed from an earlier theory proposed by Ajzen and Fishbein (1980), the Theory of Reasoned Action (TRA). The TRA was developed with the idea that humans are rational beings who weigh the outcomes of their actions before they engage in them (i.e., "reasoned action"; Ajzen & Fishbein, 1980). As a result, an underlying concept of the TRA is that behavior is determined by one's intentions to perform behavior. That is, the degree to which one is ready to behave or has determined a particular plan of action, predicts whether one will actually enact a behavior. The TRA has been used to identify factors which predict intentions (Ajzen & Fishbein, 1980). These factors are determined by beliefs about the consequences of behavior and beliefs concerning the opinions of others about the behavior. Beliefs about the consequences of behavior determine attitudes (i.e., favorable or unfavorable feelings) toward certain behaviors and normative beliefs determine subjective norms (i.e., beliefs about what others in an individual's social environment think about the behavior; Ajzen, 1985). Together, attitudes and subjective norms predict intention, which consequently predict behavior.

Although research using the framework of the TRA demonstrates some success in predicting behavioral intentions (Boyd & Wanderseman, 1991; McEachan, Taylor, Harrison, Lawton, Gardner, & Conner, 2016; Poss, 2001), the predictive ability of the TRA is limited in that it does not consider the degree of control individuals have over their ability to perform behaviors (Ajzen & Madden, 1986; Astrom & Rise, 2001; Ragin, 2011). That is to say, behavioral intentions are only relevant when a person has both external (i.e., time, opportunity, etc.) and internal (i.e., knowledge, skills, abilities, etc.) control. To address this limitation, Ajzen and colleagues (Ajzen, 1991; Ajzen & Madden, 1986) proposed adding a measure of perceived behavioral control to the model. Perceived behavioral control is defined as the degree to which individuals perceive internal and external mastery over behaviors, or more simply, whether a behavior is perceived as easy or difficult to perform (Ajzen & Madden, 1986). The revised model, which includes the perceived behavioral control construct, is known as the Theory of Planned Behavior TPB). Researchers have demonstrated the predictive ability of the TPB in varied areas of health behavior such as tobacco cessation (Murnaghan et al., 2010), condom use, (Muñoz-Silva, Sánchez-García, Nunes, & Martins,

2007), participation in disease screening programs (Cooke & French, 2008), healthy diet behaviors (Mankarious & Kothe, 2015; McDermott et al., 2015; Rich, Brandes, Mullan, & Hagger, 2015) and physical activity behaviors (Newham, Allan, Leahy-Warren, Carrick-Sen, & Alderdice, 2016; Zhang et al., 2015).

Although both the TPB and the HBM models have contributed substantially to our understanding of health behavior change, researchers have encountered limitations in being able to fully explain *why* individuals engage in health behaviors and the degree to which the models are able to explain factors like confidence or efficacy in behavior change (Mankarious & Kothe, 2015; Rich et al., 2015; Rosenstock, Strecher, & Becker, 1988). In response, some have suggested that these models may benefit from including self-regulatory factors such as self and identity.

Self and Identity

Leary and Tangney (2005) have defined the self as "the psychological apparatus that allows organisms to think consciously about themselves" (pg. 8). Identity, on the other hand, is better understood as the piece of the self that is connected to behavior (Armitage & Conner, 1999). According to identity theorists, the self is composed of multiple parts or identities. These identities are a result of social roles that have been shaped by cues in one's social environment (e.g., self as runner; Burke, 1991; Stryker, 1987; Stryker & Burke, 2000). Meaning and purpose is developed as a result of these situational selves (e.g., "runners are physical active") which then promote related behavior ("I will train for a 5K road race"). According to identity theory, greater identification with a role results in more consistent behavior that aligns with that role (Brouwer & Mosack, 2012; Stryker & Burke, 2000). As such, seeing oneself as an exerciser may engender meaning which provides the motivation needed to overcome barriers like time constraints for physical activity. For example, because an individual might identify as an exerciser, that identity may create meaning in that an exerciser is going to work out regularly. The need to affirm that identity and consequently exercise regularly is important to the self-concept of the individual. As such, the individual may make greater efforts to find time to work out despite family or occupational responsibilities, thereby maintaining the identity as an exerciser. Therefore, calling oneself an exerciser consequently creates motivation to overcome barriers.

Identity is differentiated from similar concepts such as self-schema in that identity is embedded within social roles (Stets & Burke, 2000). Schemas, on the other hand, are more cognitive in nature, representing and processing self-relevant information. Whereas identity serves as a form of self-regulatory control (e.g., the self occupies a role and the role promotes behavior), schemas are used for processing information about the self (Markus, 1977). Researchers have argued that both schemas and identity should be considered when conceptualizing behavior (Strachan & Whaley, 2013), and a recent meta-analysis on the study of schemas and identity in exercise behavior demonstrates that they are functionally the same in their relationships with other variables and correlates of behavior (Rhodes, Kaushal, & Quinlan, 2016). My focus will primarily be on identity because of its theoretical definition as the self in a social role which then corresponds with behavior. Health behavior is multidimensional and often based in goals. Therefore, identity, which has been described as a multidimensional self-concept which serves self-regulatory roles related to goal-directed behavior (Rhodes et al., 2016), will primarily be used throughout the book. However, as will be discussed in Chapter 2, the topic of interest for this book, the self-as-doer identity, embodies both identity and self-schemas.

In an effort to better understand and predict behavior change, researchers have extended both the HBM and the TPB to include self and identity components. The HBM has been extended to include self-efficacy. Rosenstock et al. (1988) argued that in the early development of the HBM, the focus of study was on relatively simple health behaviors wherein individuals likely had a good degree to confidence to perform them (e.g., immunizations). However, with the growth of the use of the model to populations such as those with chronic illness or those requiring long-term behavior changes, the need to acknowledge the role of self-efficacy within the model was established. Extending the HBM to include self-efficacy has demonstrated success in predicting health behaviors related to oral hygiene (Buglar et al., 2010), disease screenings (Norman & Brain, 2005; Noroozi, Jomand, & Tahmasebi, 2011; Sohler et al., 2015), sleep behaviors (Knowlden & Sharma, 2014), vaccination rates (Mehta, Sharma, & Lee, 2013) and healthy eating (Ferranti et al., 2014; LaBrosse & Albrecht, 2013). In general, the inclusion of self-efficacy has improved how the HBM can be used to understand health promotion behaviors.

Like the HBM, the TPB was also in need of further revisions. Researchers have argued that the weakest TPB component in predicting intentions is subjective norms (Godin & Kok, 1996; Sheppard, Hartwick, & Warshaw, 1988) and that by reorganizing subjective norms into components which reflect social influence norms (i.e., descriptive and injunctive) and self-representational norms (i.e., identity and group identification; Abraham, Sheeran, & Johnston, 1998), the TPB may be able to better explain behavior change (Astrom & Rise, 2001). In support of the hypothesis that separating out identity as a unique construct within the TPB will lead to better explanatory power for behavioral intentions, numerous researchers have found that identity can explain behavioral intentions in ways that the TPB components cannot for various health behaviors such as smoking cessation (Hassandra et al., 2011; van den Putte, Yzer, Willemsen, & de Bruijn, 2009), physical activity (Campbell & Sheeran, 2001; Leyland, van Wersch, & Woodhouse, 2014; Thompson & Rise, 2002), and diet behaviors (Brouwer & Mosack, 2015; Armitage & Conner, 1999; Sparks & Guthrie, 1998). Others have determined that identity is one of the most important predictors of behaviors and intentions and theoretically fits well into the TPB model (Rise, Sheeran, & Hukkelberg, 2010). Rise and colleagues (2010) have also distinguished identity from past behaviors, group identity, and the other components in the TPB, leading to the conclusion that there is sufficient evidence for identity to be added as a variable to the TPB model.

Overall, self and identity have been meaningful factors in predicting health behaviors. That both have successfully been added to existing health behavior theories and have demonstrated success in predicting diverse health behaviors supports the idea that such factors can be conceptualized as unique constructs which provide explanatory power for both intentions to perform behaviors and actual behavioral enactment. Furthermore, the degree to which self and identity have provided additional explanatory power in health behavior change also supports their use in intervention development aimed at modifying health behaviors.

Conclusion

In sum, health is a multidimensional construct requiring comprehensive approaches to health promotion. Many of the health maladies that individuals face can be modified if health-diminishing behaviors are reduced and health promoting behaviors are increased. Existing health theories such as the TPB and the HBM have been fundamental in developing an understanding how social and psychological factors influence health behavior change. Moreover, the addition of self and identity to these models have demonstrated even greater promise for predicting and modifying health behavior. Although there is great value in adding self and identity to the study of health behavior, changes to lifestyle behaviors also require motivation, especially to overcome many of the idiosyncratic and contextual barriers that individuals face. A construct that embodies the self, identity, and motivation, and that which is the primary topic of this book, is the self-as-doer identity (Houser-Marko & Sheldon, 2006).

In the next several chapters, I will discuss how the self-as-doer identity accounts for motivation and can be incorporated into health behavior change efforts (Chapter 2 and Chapter 3). Research and recommendations for how the self-as-doer can be used in both non-clinical (Chapter 4) and clinical (Chapter 5) populations will be discussed; and the role that a self-as-doer identity can play in various research and clinical settings in the promotion and maintenance of health behavior change will be the concluding topic in this book (Chapter 6). Research providing evidence for the self-as-doer is ongoing. As such, existing research and the implications of the findings and generalizations to other populations will be reviewed because of the potential to inform existing health promotion programs. This book has been written in such a way as to appeal to diverse audiences interested in health behavior change and maintenance. However, health care professionals and non-scientists may be particularly interested in chapters discussing the usability and applicability of the self-as-doer in various populations (e.g., Chapters 4, 5, and 6). Those working in clinical and research settings might be specifically interested in chapters describing the development and measurement of the self-as-doer identity (Chapter 3), outcomes of an intervention for the self-as-doer identity (e.g., Chapter 4), and recommendations for its use in other research and clinical contexts (Chapter 6).

References

Abraham, C., Sheeran, P., & Johnston, M. (1998). From health beliefs to self-regulation: Theoretical advances in the psychology of action control. *Psychology and Health, 13*, 569–591. doi: 10.1080/08870449808407420

Agboola, S., Mcneill, A., Coleman, T., & Leonardi Bee, J. (2010). A systematic review of the effectiveness of smoking relapse prevention interventions for abstinent smokers. *Addiction, 105*, 1362–1380. doi: 10.1111/j.1360–0443.2010.02996.x

Ajzen, I. (1985). From intentions to action: A theory of planned behavior. In K. Kuhland, & J. Beckman (Eds.), *Action control: From cognition to behavior* (pp. 11–39). Heidelberg: Springer.

Ajzen, I. (1991). The theory of planned behavior. *Organizational Behavior and Human Decision Processes, 50*, 179–211. Retrieved from http://people.umass.edu/psyc661/pdf/tpb.obhdp.pdf

Ajzen, I., & Fishbein, M. (1980). *Understanding attitudes and predicting social behavior*. Englewood Cliffs, NJ: Prentice-Hall.

Ajzen, I., & Madden, T. J. (1986). Prediction of goal-directed behavior: Attitudes, intentions and perceived behavioral control. *Journal of Experimental Social Psychology, 22*, 453–474. doi: 10.1016/0022–1031(86)90045–4

Anagnostopoulos, F., Buchanan, H., Frousiounioti, S., Niakas, D., & Potamianos, G. (2011). Self-efficacy and oral hygiene beliefs about toothbrushing in dental patients: A model-guided study. *Behavioral Medicine, 37*(4), 132–139. doi: 10.1080/08964289.2011.636770

Armitage, C. J., & Conner, M. (1999). Distinguishing perceptions of control from self-efficacy: Predicting consumption of a low-fat diet using the theory of planned behavior. *Journal of Applied Social Psychology, 29*, 72–90. doi: 10.1111/j.1559–1816.1999.tb01375.x

Asare, M., Sharma, M., Bernard, A. L., Rojas-Guyler, L., & Wang, L. L. (2013). Using the health belief model to determine safer sexual behavior among African immigrants. *Journal of Health Care for the Poor and Underserved, 24*(1), 120–134. doi: 10.1353/hpu.2013.0020

Astrom, A. N., & Rise, J. (2001). Young adults' intentions to eat healthy good: Extending the theory of planned behavior. *Psychology and Health, 16*, 223–237. doi: 10.1080/08870440108405501

Avenell, A., Broom, J., Brown, T. J., Poobalan, A., Aucott, L., Stearns, S. C., . . . Grant, A. M. (2004). Systematic review of the long-term effects and economic consequences of treatments for obesity and implications for health improvement. *Health Technology Assessment, 8*(21), 1–182. Retrieved from www.ncbi.nlm.nih. gov/pubmedhealth/PMH0015087/pdf/PubMedHealth_PMH0015087.pdf

Bouma, A. J., van Wilgen, P., & Dijkstra, A. (2015). The barrier-belief approach in the counseling of physical activity. *Patient Education and Counseling, 98(2), 129–136. doi: 10.1016/j.pec.2014.10.003*

Boyd, B., & Wanderseman, A. (1991). Predicting undergraduate condom use with the Fishbein and Azjen and the Triandis attitude-behavior models: Implications for public health intervention. *Journal for Applied Social Psychology, 21*, 1810–1830. doi: 10.1111/j.1559-1816.1991.tb00506.x

Brenner, A. T., Ko, L. K., Janz, N., Gupta, S., & Inadomi, J. (2015). Race/ethnicity and primary language: Health beliefs about colorectal cancer screening in a diverse, low-income population. *Journal of Health Care for the Poor and Underserved, 26*(3), 824–838.

Brouwer, A. M., & Mosack, K. E. (2012). "I am a blood sugar checker": Intervening effects of the self-as-doer identity on the relationship between self-efficacy and diabetes self-care behaviors. *Self and Identity, 11*, 472–491. doi: 10.1080/15298868.2011.603901

Brouwer, A. M., & Mosack, K. E. (2015). Expanding the theory of planned behavior to predict healthy eating behaviors: Exploring the role of a healthy eater identity. *Nutrition and Food Science, 45*, 39–53. doi: 0.1108/NFS-06-2014-0055

Buglar, M. E., White, K. M., & Robinson, N. G. (2010). The role of self-efficacy in dental patients' brushing and flossing: Testing an extended health belief model. *Patient Education and Counseling, 78*(2), 269–272. doi: 10.1016/j.pec.2009.06.014

Burke, P. J. (1991). An identity theory approach to commitment. *Social Psychology Quarterly, 54*, 239–251. Retrieved from www.jstor.org/stable/2786653

Campbell, S., & Sheeran, P. (2001). *Self-identity and exercise*. Unpublished raw data, University of Sheffield, UK.

Center for Disease Control (2014). *Facts about physical activity*. Retrieved from www.cdc.gov/physicalactivity/data/facts.htm

Center for Disease Control (2015a). *Annual number (in Thousands) of new cases of diagnosed diabetes among adults aged 18–79 years, United States, 1980–2014.* Retrieved from www.cdc.gov/diabetes/statistics/incidence/fig1.htm

Center for Disease Control (2015b). *Lifestyle risk factors*. Retrieved from https:// ephtracking.cdc.gov/showLifestyleRiskFactorsMain.action

Cooke, R., & French, D. P. (2008). How well do the theory of reasoned action and theory of planned behaviour predict intentions and attendance at screening programmes? A meta-analysis. *Psychology & Health, 23*(7), 745–765. doi: 10.1080/08870440701544437

Crutzen, R., Viechtbauer, W., Spigt, M., & Kotz, D. (2015). Differential attrition in health behaviour change trials: A systematic review and meta-analysis. *Psychology & Health, 30*(1), 122–134. doi: 10.1080/08870446.2014.953526

de Bruin, M., McCambridge, J., & Prins, J. M. (2015). Reducing the risk of bias in health behaviour change trials: Improving trial design, reporting or bias assessment criteria? A review and case study. *Psychology & Health, 30*(1), 8–34. doi: 10.1080/08870446.2014.953531

Deshpande, S., Basil, M. D., & Basil, D. Z. (2009). Factors influencing healthy eating habits among college students: An application of the health belief model. *Health Marketing Quarterly, 26*(2), 145–164. doi: 10.1080/07359680802619834

Dombrowski, S. U., Knittle, K., Avenell, A., Araujo-Soares, V., & Sniehotta, F. F. (2014). Long-term maintenance of weight loss in obese adults: A systematic review of randomised controlled trials of nonsurgical weight loss maintenance interventions with meta-analyses. *British Medical Journal, 348*, g2646. doi: 10.1136/bmj.g2646

Dumville, J. C., Torgerson, D., & Hewitt, C. E. (2006). Reporting attrition in randomised controlled trials. *BMJ: British Medical Journal, 332*(7547), 969–971. Retrieved from www.bmj.com/content/332/7547/969

Ferranti, E. P., Narayan, K. V., Reilly, C. M., Foster, J., McCullough, M., Ziegler, T. R., . . . Dunbar, S. B. (2014). Dietary self-efficacy predicts AHEI diet quality in women with previous gestational diabetes. *Diabetes Educator, 40*(5), 688–699. doi: 10.1177/0145721714539735

Fishbein, M. (2002). The role of theory in HIV prevention. In D. F. Marks (Ed.), *The health psychology reader* (pp. 120–126). London: Sage.

Ford, E. S., Zhao, G., Tsai, J., & Li, C. (2011). Low-risk lifestyle behaviors and all-cause mortality: Findings from the National Health and Nutrition Examination Survey III Mortality Study. *American Journal of Public Health, 101*(10), 1922–1929. doi: 10.2105/AJPH.2011.300167

Foster, G. D., Wyatt, H. R., Hill, J. O., Makris, A. P., Rosenbaum, D. L., Brill, C., . . . Klein, S. (2010). Weight and metabolic outcomes after 2 years on a low-carbohydrate versus low-fat diet: A randomized trial. *Annals of Internal Medicine, 153*, 147–157. doi: 10.7326/0003-4819-153-3-201008030-00005

Fryar, C. D., Carroll, M. D., & Ogden, C. L. (2016). Prevalence of overweight, obesity and extreme obesity among adults aged 20 and over: United States, 1960–1962 through 2013–2014. *National Center for Health Statistics Health E-Stats*, Retrieved from www.cdc.gov/nchs/data/hestat/obesity_adult_13_14/obesity_adult_13_14.pdf

Godin, G., & Kok, G. (1996). The theory of planned behavior: A review of its applications to health-related behaviors. *American Journal of Health Promotion, 11*, 87–98. doi: 10.4278/0890-1171-11.2.87

Hamel, L. M., & Robbins, L. B. (2013). Computer-and web-based interventions to promote healthy eating among children and adolescents: A systematic review. *Journal of Advanced Nursing, 69*(1), 16–30. doi: 10.1111/j.1365-2648.2012.06086.x

Hassandra, M., Vlachopoulos, S. P., Kosmidou, E., Hatzigeorgiadis, A., Goudas, M., & Theodorakis, Y. (2011). Predicting students' intention to smoke by theory of planned behaviour variables and parental influences across school grade levels. *Psychology & Health, 26*(9), 1241–1258. doi: 10.1080/08870446.2011.605137

Hastert, T. A., Ruterbusch, J. J., Beresford, S. A., Sheppard, L., & White, E. (2016). Contribution of health behaviors to the association between area-level socioeconomic status and cancer mortality. *Social Science & Medicine, 148*, 52–58. doi: 10.1016/j.socscimed.2015.11.023

Houser-Marko, L., & Sheldon, K. M. (2006). Motivating behavioral persistence: The self-as-doer construct. *Personality and Social Psychology Bulletin, 32*, 1037–1049. doi: 10.1177/0146167206287974

Jones, C. J., Smith, H., & Llewellyn, C. (2014). Evaluating the effectiveness of health belief model interventions in improving adherence: A systematic review. *Health Psychology Review, 8*(3), 253–269. doi: 10.1080/17437199.2013.802623

Kelly, S., Martin, S., Kuhn, I., Cowan, A., Brayne, C., & Lafortune, L. (2016). Barriers and facilitators to the uptake and maintenance of healthy behaviours by people at mid-life: A rapid systematic review. *PLoS One, 11*(1), e0145074. doi: 10.1371/journal.pone.0145074

Kimmons, J., Gillespie, C., Seymour, J., Serdula, M., & Blanck, H. M. (2009). Fruit and vegetable intake among adolescents and adults in the United States: Percentage meeting individual recommendations. *Medscape Journal of Medicine, 11*, 26. Retrieved from www.ncbi.nlm.nih.gov/pmc/articles/PMC2654704/?tool=pubmed

Knowlden, A. P., & Sharma, M. (2014). Health belief structural equation model predicting sleep behavior of employed college students. *Family & Community Health: The Journal of Health Promotion & Maintenance, 37*(4), 271–278. doi: 10.1097/FCH.0000000000000043

LaBrosse, L., & Albrecht, J. A. (2013). Pilot intervention with adolescents to increase knowledge and consumption of folate-rich foods based on the Health Belief Model. *International Journal of Consumer Studies, 37*(3), 271–278. doi: 10.1111/ijcs.12004

Leary, M. R., & Tangney, J. P. (2005). The self as an organizing construct in the behavioral and social sciences. In M. R. Leary, & J. P. Tangney (Eds.), *Handbook of self and identity* (pp. 3–14). New York: The Guilford Press.

Lee, H., Stange, M., & Ahluwalia, J. (2015). Breast cancer screening behaviors among Korean American immigrant women: Findings from the health belief model. *Journal of Transcultural Nursing, 26*, 450–457.

Lee Olstad, D., Ball, K., Abbott, G., McNaughton, S. A., Le, H. D., Ni Mhurchu, C., . . . Crawford, D. A. (2016). A process evaluation of the Supermarket Healthy Eating for Life (SHELf) randomized controlled trial. *International Journal of Behavioral Nutrition and Physical Activity, 13*, 2–15. doi: 10.1186/s12966-016-0352-3

Leyland, S. D., van Wersch, A., & Woodhouse, D. (2014). Testing an extended theory of planned behaviour to predict intention to participate in health-related exercise during long-distance flight travel. *International Journal of Sport and Exercise Psychology, 12*(1), 34–48. doi: 10.1080/1612197X.2012.756255

Loef, M., & Walach, H. (2012). The combined effects of healthy lifestyle behaviors on all cause mortality: A systematic review and meta-analysis. *Preventive*

Medicine: An International Journal Devoted to Practice and Theory, 55(3), 163–170. doi: 10.1016/j.ypmed.2012.06.017

Mankarious, E., & Kothe, E. (2015). A meta-analysis of the effects of measuring theory of planned behaviour constructs on behaviour within prospective studies. *Health Psychology Review, 9*(2), 190–204. doi: 10.1080/17437199.2014.927722

Markus, H. (1977). Self-schemata and processing information about the self. *Journal of Personality and Social Psychology, 35*, 63–78. doi: 10.1037/0022–3514.35.2.63

Martinez, D. J., Turner, M. M., Pratt-Chapman, M., Kashima, K., Hargreaves, M. K., Dignan, M. B., & Hébert, J. R. (2016). The effect of changes in health beliefs among African-American and rural white church congregants enrolled in an obesity intervention: A qualitative evaluation. *Journal of Community Health: The Publication for Health Promotion and Disease Prevention, 41*, 518–525. doi: 10.1007/s10900–015–0125-y

McDermott, M. S., Oliver, M., Simnadis, T., Beck, E. J., Coltman, T., Iverson, D., . . . Sharma, R. (2015). The theory of planned behaviour and dietary patterns: A systematic review and meta-analysis. *Preventive Medicine: An International Journal Devoted to Practice and Theory, 81*, 150–156.

McEachan, R., Taylor, N., Harrison, R., Lawton, R., Gardner, P., & Conner, M. (2016). Meta-analysis of the reasoned action approach (RAA) to understanding health behaviors. *Annals of Behavioral Medicine, 50*(4), 592–612. doi: 10.1007/s12160-016-9798-4

Mehta, P., Sharma, M., & Lee, R. C. (2013). Designing and evaluating a health belief model-based intervention to increase intent of HPV vaccination among college males. *International Quarterly of Community Health Education, 34*(1), 101–117. doi: 10.2190/IQ.34.1.h

Moore, L. V., & Thompson, F. E. (2015). Adults meeting fruit and vegetable intake recommendations—United States, 2013. *Morbidity and Mortality Weekly Report, 64*, 709–713. Retrieved from www.cdc.gov/mmwr/preview/mmwrhtml/mm6426a1.htm

Muñoz-Silva, A., Sánchez-García, M., Nunes, C., & Martins, A. (2007). Gender differences in condom use prediction with theory of reasoned action and planned behaviour: The role of self-efficacy and control. *AIDS Care, 19*, 1177–1181. doi: 10.1080/09540120701402772

Murnaghan, D. A., Blanchard, C. M., Rodgers, W. M., LaRosa, J. N., MacQuarrie, C. R., MacLellan, D. L., & Gray, B. (2010). Predictors of physical activity, healthy eating and being smoke-free in teens: A theory of planned behaviour approach. *Psychology and Health, 25*, 925–941. doi: 10.1080/0887044092866894

Near, S. M., & Zimmerman, R. S. (2005). Health behavior theory and cumulative knowledge regarding health behaviors: Are we moving in the right direction? *Health Education Research, 20*, 275–290. doi: 10.1093/her/cyg113

Newham, J. J., Allan, C., Leahy-Warren, P., Carrick-Sen, D., & Alderdice, F. (2016). Intentions toward physical activity and resting behavior in pregnant women: Using the theory of planned behavior framework in a cross-sectional study. *Birth: Issues in Perinatal Care, 43*(1), 49–57. doi: 10.1111/birt.12211

Norman, P., & Brain, K. (2005). An application of an extended health belief model to the prediction of breast self-examination among women with a family history of breast cancer. *British Journal of Health Psychology, 10*(1), 1–16. doi: 10.1348/135910704X24752

Noroozi, A., Jomand, T., & Tahmasebi, R. (2011). Determinants of breast self-examination performance among Iranian women: An application of the Health Belief Model. *Journal of Cancer Education, 26*(2), 365–374. doi: 10.1007/s13187-010-0158-y

Poss, J. E. (2001). Developing a new model for cross-cultural research: Synthesizing the Health Belief Model and the Theory of Reasoned Action. *Advances in Nursing Science, 23*, 1–15. doi: 10.1097/00012272-200106000-00002

Prapavessis, H., Jesus, S., Fitzgeorge, L., Faulkner, G., Maddison, R., & Batten, S. (2016). Exercise to enhance smoking cessation: The getting physical on cigarette randomized control trial. *Annals of Behavioral Medicine, 50*(3), 358–369. doi: 10.1007/s12160-015-9761-9

Ragin, D. F. (2011). *Health psychology: An interdisciplinary approach to health.* Boston: Prentice Hall.

Rhodes, R. E., Kaushal, N., & Quinlan, A. (2016). Is physical activity a part of who I am? A review and meta-analysis of identity, schema and physical activity. *Health Psychology Review, 10*(2), 204–225. doi: 10.1080/17437199.2016.1143334

Rich, A., Brandes, K., Mullan, B., & Hagger, M. (2015). Theory of planned behavior and adherence in chronic illness: A meta-analysis. *Journal of Behavioral Medicine, 38*(4), 673–688. doi: 10.1007/s10865-015-9644-3

Riekert, K. A., Ockene, J. K., & Pbert, L. (Eds.). (2014). *The handbook of health behavior change.* New York: Springer Publishing.

Rise, J., Sheeran, P., & Hukkelberg, S. (2010). The role of self-identity in the theory of planned behavior: A meta-analysis. *Journal of Applied Social Psychology, 40*, 1085–1105. doi: 10.1111/j.1559-1816.2010.00611.x/pdf

Rosenstock, I. M. (1974). Historical origins of the health belief model. *Health Education Monographs, 2*, 1–8.

Rosenstock, I. M. (1990). The health belief model: Explaining health behavior through expectancies. In K. Glanz, F. M. Lewis, B. K. Rimer, K. Glanz, F. M. Lewis, & B. K. Rimer (Eds.), *Health behavior and health education: Theory, research, and practice* (pp. 39–62). San Francisco, CA: Jossey-Bass.

Rosenstock, I. M., Strecher, V. J., & Becker, M. H. (1988). Social learning theory and the Health Belief Model. *Health Education Quarterly, 15*(2), 175–183. doi: 10.1177/109019818801500203

Sapp, S. G., & Weng, C. (2007). Examination of the health-belief model to predict the dietary quality and body mass of adults. *International Journal of Consumer Studies, 31*(3), 189–194. doi: 10.1111/j.1470-6431.2006.00500.x

Sheppard, B. H., Hartwick, J., & Warshaw, P. R. (1988). The theory of reasoned action: A meta-analysis of past research with recommendations for modifications and future research. *Journal of Consumer Research, 15*(3), 325–343. doi: 10.1086/209170

Sohler, N. L., Jerant, A., & Franks, P. (2015). Socio-psychological factors in the Expanded Health Belief Model and subsequent colorectal cancer screening. *Patient Education and Counseling, 98*(7), 901–907. doi: 10.1016/j.pec.2015.03.023

Sparks, P., & Guthrie, C. (1998). Self-identity and the theory of planned behavior: Useful addition or unhelpful artifice? *Journal of Applied Social Psychology, 28,* 1393–1410. doi: 10.1111/j.1559-1816.1998.tb01683.x

Spohr, S. A., Nandy, R., Gandhiraj, D., Vemulapalli, A., Anne, S., & Walters, S. T. (2015). Efficacy of SMS text message interventions for smoking cessation: A meta-analysis. *Journal of Substance Abuse Treatment, 56,* 1–10. doi: 10.1016/j.jsat.2015.01.011

Spruijt-Metz, D., Hekler, E., Saranummi, N., Intille, S., Korhonen, I., Nilsen, W., . . . Pavel, M. (2015). Building new computational models to support health behavior change and maintenance: New opportunities in behavioral research. *Translational Behavioral Medicine, 5*(3), 335–346. doi: 10.1007/s13142-015-0324-1

Stets, J. E., & Burke, P. J. (2000). Identity theory and social identity theory. *Social Psychology Quarterly, 63,* 224–237. Retrieved from http://wat2146.ucr.edu/papers/00a.pdf

Strachan, S. M., & Whaley, D. E. (2013). Identities, schemas, and definitions: How aspects of the self influence exercise behavior. In P. Ekkekakis, D. B. Cook, L. L. Craft, S. N. Culos-Reed, J. L. Etnier, M. Hamer, . . . M. Ussher (Eds.), *Routledge handbook of physical activity and mental health* (pp. 212–223). New York: Routledge/Taylor & Francis Group.

Stryker, S. (1987). Identity theory: Development and extensions. In K. Yardley, & T. Honess (Eds.), *Self and identity: Psychosocial perspectives* (pp. 89–103). London: John Wiley.

Stryker, S., & Burke, P. J. (2000). The past, present, and future of identity theory. *Social Psychology Quarterly, 63,* 284–297. Retrieved from www.jstor.org/stable/2695840

Thompson, M., & Rise, J. (2002). *The theory of planned behavior extended: The role of past behavior and social influence.* Unpublished manuscript.

van den Putte, B., Yzer, M., Willemsen, M. C., & de Bruijn, G. (2009). The effects of smoking self-identity and quitting self-identity on attempts to quit smoking. *Health Psychology, 28*(5), 535–544. doi: 10.1037/a0015199

Weissman, J., Pratt, L. A., Miller, E. A., & Parker, J. D. (2015). *Serious psychological distress among adults: United States, 2009–2013.* (NCHS data brief No. 203). Retrieved from Center for Disease Control website: www.cdc.gov/nchs/data/databriefs/db203.pdf

World Health Organization (1948). *Constitution of WHO: Principles.* Retrieved from www.who.int/about/mission/en/

Wright, P. J., Randall, A. K., & Hayes, J. G. (2012). Predicting the condom assertiveness of collegiate females in the United States from the expanded health belief model. *International Journal of Sexual Health, 24*(2), 137–153. doi: 10.1080/19317611.2012.661396

Zhang, N., Campo, S., Yang, J., Janz, K. F., Snetselaar, L. G., & Eckler, P. (2015). Effects of social support about physical activity on social networking sites: Applying the theory of planned behavior. *Health Communication, 30*(12), 1277–1285. doi: 10.1080/10410236.2014.940669

2 The Self-as-Doer

An Introduction

Amanda M. Brouwer and
Linda S. Houser-Marko

The self-as-doer is a self-schema (i.e., a way of cognitively representing the self; Markus & Wurf, 1987) where behavior and identity are linked in working memory. The self-as-doer describes individuals in terms of their identification with *doing* a behavior (i.e., an exerciser, a vegetable eater, a good grade getter; Brouwer & Mosack, 2015; Houser-Marko & Sheldon, 2006). It is focused on present action, is dynamic, and develops from self-feedback. Furthermore, it represents enacting a behavior instead of the enjoyment of that behavior. As will be discussed in this chapter, the self-as-doer can be a source of motivation for various behaviors in that the degree to which one identifies with doing a behavior serves as a motivational resource for engaging in that behavior. As a motivational construct that goes beyond self-concordance, commitment, or expectancy (Houser-Marko & Sheldon, 2006), the self-as-doer can then be applied to activities and behaviors that might not be inherently enjoyable, such as practicing the piano, going for a jog, or engaging in aversive health behaviors. Furthermore, doer-identification predicts goal persistence and effort and has been shown to exist as an ongoing or recurrent self-schema. Researchers have also been able to "activate" a self-as-doer identity by increasing it momentarily (Houser-Marko & Sheldon, 2006). Given the focus on motivation and that the self-as-doer can be "activated," it is a promising application to health behavior change.

The self-as-doer is rooted within identity theory. Identity theory defines identity as seeing oneself as the occupant of a role. Often that role is situated within a highly diverse environment which, in turn, shapes the self (Stets & Burke, 2000). In the process of development, as the person begins to take on multiple roles put forth by the social surroundings, one's identity develops and the self begins to occupy various roles. Throughout the process of developing identity and occupying roles, the individual internalizes meanings and expectations associated with that role. That is to say, it is a recursive process. Furthermore as meaning for each role is developed, an identity associated with that role also continues to develop. Then, the social standards and qualifications of the understood role guide the individual's behaviors (Stets & Burke, 2000).

Consider as an example the "self-as-parent" role. A man has a child. His role becomes defined by his social and emotional environment, his child and others around him. The parent then considers the meaning and expectations involved in such a role: he must provide for the child's required physical needs (e.g., shelter, food) and the emotional expectations (i.e., to love, care for, and discipline his child). The acceptance and personalization of these expectations then guide his behaviors in the "self-as-parent" role; he purchases blankets, food, toys; provides love and affection; and protects the child from harm. This "self-as-parent" identity guides his behavior, which then supports his identity and consequently feeds back to engaging in more of the "self-as-parent" behavior. The more central one's identity is to oneself, the greater the chance that a person will behave in a way that supports that identity (Stets & Burke, 2000). Research supports these postulations especially for health behaviors. For example, Strachan and Brawley (2008, 2009) found that when people identified as exercisers or healthy eaters they were more likely to exercise or make healthy diet choices than those who did not identify as such.

The self-as-doer differs from identity theory in that it can vary on how important, desired, or central the identity is to the person. In other words, a self-as-doer identity may be more or less integrated into one's self-concept, but can still serve as a motivational resource for behavior. Consider, for example, an individual with a self-as-doer identity of "exerciser." If this individual is taking up a new exercise plan he may view himself as an "exerciser," but this identity may not yet be a central identity, an identity that is strongly connected to the self-concept. However, over time and as the result of ongoing feedback, the "exerciser" self-as-doer identity may become more central to his self-concept. According to self-as-doer theory, in both circumstances, it is the link between the behavior and the identity that motivates behavior, not just the degree to which one identifies as an "exerciser." Thus, seeing oneself as the *doer* of the behavior is what creates motivation for behavior.

The self-as-doer can also be thought of as an identity linkage, similar to the linkages in the triangle model of responsibility (Schlenker, Britt, Pennington, Murphy, & Doherty, 1994; Schlenker, Pontari, & Christopher, 2001). The triangle model suggests that behavior can be determined, in part, by the social rules that affect behavior in a given context (i.e., prescriptions) and the degree to which one's identity is linked with those prescriptions (i.e., identity images), which is one side of the triangle (Schlenker et al., 1994). Consider, for example, an individual who joins a gym. The prescriptions of the gym context are such that individuals go there to work out, attend fitness classes, or lift weights. If a person strongly endorses an identity relevant to the context of being a member of a gym, that individual is more likely to behave in accordance with the prescribed rules of the social context. That is to say, this individual may be more likely to work out regularly and attend fitness classes because she is part of the gym context (that includes prescriptions for behavior) and an individual whose identity image is aligned with the context must adhere to those rules in order to maintain the identity image. As such, the linkage between one's identity image and the prescriptions of a context can promote behavior with stronger connections eliciting more consistent and frequent behavior (Schlenker et al., 1994). The self-as-doer is similar because of the identity linkage. However, instead of an identity-prescription linkage, the self-as-doer construct is an identity-behavior linkage.

Houser-Marko and Sheldon (2006) used this framework to describe the self-as-doer: one's identity or self-schema can be linked to a certain behavior just as identity can be linked with social prescriptions. The link between identity and behavior then creates the self-as-doer identity which serves as a source of motivation for behavioral engagement. *Such as "I do this, I am a doer, so I will do this again."* For example, one may have the goal to exercise more frequently. When this goal is linked with an exerciser identity, one now sees him or herself as the doer of that behavior, a frequent exerciser. This identity has certain behavioral expectations or rules that govern behavior. For example, to be a frequent exerciser one needs to engage in physical activity on a regular basis, perhaps purchase exercise equipment, or clothes that will facilitate exercising frequently. By endorsing the identity as the doer of one's behavior, one is linking the identity image with the behaviors in a way that seeing oneself as the doer motivates one to follow the established rules and expectations for corresponding behaviors.

Taken together, identity theory and the triangle model of responsibility suggest that if personal identity is connected with social principles, ideals, and expectations, then this identity will encourage behavior in accordance with those principles and ideals. Additionally, it is more likely that behavior will occur and continue to occur if the person is closely identified with the action or behavior. In accordance with these theories, the self-as-doer theory draws a link between identity and behavior, suggesting that the more one identifies with a goal or behavior, the more likely one is to participate in related behavior. A key point is that one behaves in accordance with his or her identity *because* that individual defines him or herself as a *doer* of the behavior. The self-as-doer was initially conceptualized by transforming a particular goal (i.e., to walk daily) into an active representation of an agent performing a behavior (i.e., daily walker). The conceptualization of a daily walker, which represents one's identity aligned with its social principles and ideals (i.e., daily walkers walk; they have walking shoes and perhaps walking friends that walk at a lunch break or after work; walkers are healthy and happy individuals; etc.) promotes behavior corresponding to that identity. For example, a man with diabetes might have a goal of checking his blood glucose regularly; if he considers the goal in doer-terms, he might then be more inclined to see himself as a blood glucose checker, the *doer* of the behavior, and therefore be more likely to check his blood glucose. The self-as-doer capitalizes on not only the identification of one's identity role, but the behavior based upon that role. The ability to connect identity and behavior to provide an additional source of motivation to encourage both the instigation and maintenance of behavior change is what makes the self-as-doer unique.

Attributes of the Self-as-Doer

There are several unique attributes of the self-as-doer that distinguish it from other motivational theories which, we argue, make it a superior theory on which to base health behavior change interventions. Work on the self-as-doer by Houser-Marko and Sheldon (2006) and others (e.g., Brouwer & Mosack, 2012, 2013, 2015) has established that the self-as-doer can be defined across identity domains. Likewise, the self-as-doer can be domain-general or domain-specific. Either form has been shown to predict behavior, although domain-specific forms tend to be better predictors of domain-specific behaviors. For example, Houser-Marko and Sheldon (2006) found that both a general self-as-doer identity (i.e., identity as the doer of several diverse behavioral goals) and an academic-specific self-as-doer identity (i.e., identity formed specifically from academic goals) were predictors of grade point averages (GPAs) of college students more than three years later. The academic-specific doer-identity was, however, a better predictor of academic success than the domain-general doer identity. The self-as-doer also has the capacity to be defined in terms of the self as a whole ("dedicated worker") or the self as a specific process ("good grade getter"). This attribute contributes to its ability to be used in promoting both general health behaviors (e.g., "healthy eater") and specific behavioral regimens like those for individuals with chronic illness (e.g., "medication taker"; Brouwer & Mosack, 2013).

A second attribute is that the self-as-doer is a dynamic agent, focused on engaging in behavior in the present rather than a representation of past behavior. As noted earlier, Houser-Marko and Sheldon (2006) theorized that the self-as-doer is the identification with *doing* a behavior and therefore should be associated with the present process of striving for one's goal (i.e., process identification) rather than goal achievement or previously accomplished behaviors. These theoretical underpinnings were supported by a series of studies demonstrating that the self-as-doer predicted process identification and exercise behaviors regardless of a person's experience with previous exercise goals (Houser-Marko & Sheldon, 2006). This finding is important because it suggests that there is a unique contribution that the process of developing self-as-doer identities has above and beyond the common process of making behavioral goals. This attribute of the self-as-doer is what makes it distinct from other motivational theories. That is to say, because the self-as-doer is a dynamic agent focused on behavioral engagement in the present, the focus of the individual is to perform the behavior, to *do* the behavior, rather than to enjoy the behavior or be rewarded by it. As such, the self-as-doer can be a source of motivation for health behaviors that are not necessarily inherently reinforcing. For example, taking medication among people living with diabetes might not be inherently reinforcing, but changing the focus of the behavior to be on the present behavior, as is done with self-as-doer identity, takes away the need for a reward or fear of aversive outcomes (e.g., taking medication that has unpleasant side effects; Brouwer & Mosack, 2013; Houser-Marko & Sheldon, 2006).

Thirdly, the self-as-doer identity can be applied and "activated" in multiple ways. Researchers have demonstrated that individuals can think of the self-as-doer either momentarily or recurrently. In support of how the self-as-doer can be activated or accessible over time, Houser-Marko and Sheldon (2006) recorded academic goals and doer-identities of college freshmen and then assessed their level of academic success three and a half years later. They found that students remembered their previously established educational goals better when they had stronger self-as-doer identities and that greater doer-identification predicted higher GPAs. The authors concluded that not only did the self-as-doer identity have predictive power for future behavioral outcomes, but that a doer-identity was an "enduring and chronically salient part of the self" for those students (p. 1047).

Further, the doer-identity can be made accessible even for individuals who do not already consider themselves as the doer of their behaviors. To demonstrate how the self-as-doer could be activated momentarily, Houser-Marko and Sheldon (2006) had participants complete a task intended to elicit a general self-as-doer identity by having them read a story about persistence (i.e., *The Little Engine that Could*) and write an essay on how the lesson of persistence applied to themselves. The researchers then compared the self-as-doer priming condition to three other conditions, wherein (1) individuals read the same story on persistence and wrote an essay on how that story applied to another person, (2) they read a story not meant to elicit persistence (i.e., *Curious George*) and wrote an essay applying the moral of the story to themselves or (3) read *Curious George* and applied the moral to another person. They found that those who were primed for the self-as-doer identity and applied it to themselves persisted longer at a subsequent exercise task than those in the other three groups. From these research findings, the authors concluded that self-as-doer identity can be activated momentarily via a prime where the concept was applied or linked to the self, and also that it can be activated for those who do not already see themselves as doers.

The fact that there were no significant effects for the condition in which participants read the persistence story and applied the moral of the story to others also suggests that self-as-doer identity is effective as an identity orientation that is focused on the self rather than on others. That the authors found that the self-as-doer identity is an internal source of motivation focused on the self and one that can be activated even for those who do not already possess the identity, theoretically strengthens the ability of the self-as-doer to enact and sustain health behavior changes because it reduces outside interference and can be applied to those who have not yet begun changes in health behaviors. The findings from this research also support the identity-linkage concept from the triangle model of responsibility (Schlenker et al., 2001) in that the doer-identity only had effects when both the self and behavior were linked. As such, it is not just the self that promotes persistence, but that the conceptualization of the self has been associated with behavior (Houser-Marko & Sheldon, 2006).

Given the relatively flexible and versatile nature of the self-as-doer, its application to increase health behaviors and psychological well-being is potentially widespread. Researchers have used the self-as-doer construct in a variety of research domains including general health behaviors such as physical activity (Brouwer, n.d.; Brouwer & Mosack, 2013; Houser-Marko & Sheldon, 2006) and diet (Brouwer & Mosack, 2015) and with disease-specific behaviors such as diabetes self-care behaviors (Brouwer & Mosack, 2012, 2013). Others have examined the degree to which self-as-doer identities are related to social support and social identity in an effort to promote greater adjustment and well-being among individuals with acquired brain injuries (Walsh, Muldoon, Gallagher, & Fortune, 2015). As will be discussed in subsequent chapters, the self-as-doer identity has had success in predicting, activating, and maintaining health behavior change.

Overall, research on the self-as-doer identity demonstrates that the doer construct is a dynamic identity, rooted in identity theory, which motivates behavior change through its ability to link one's identity with behavior. It can be developed to describe the self as a whole or be domain-specific. As has been summarized elsewhere, the self-as-doer identity "focuses on present behavior rather than outcome expectancies, performing behaviors rather than enjoying them, and demonstrating one's identity to oneself rather than demonstrating a socially acceptable identity to others" (Brouwer & Mosack, 2012, p. 3) . Finally, it is versatile in its use, having already been success-fully applied to both general and specific health-related behaviors.

Differences Between the Self-as-Doer and Existing Motivation and Health Theories

In order to determine the unique contribution of the self-as-doer among existing motivational and health theories, it is important to assess how the self-as-doer is different from related motivation and identity theories that have been found to be influential in health behavior outcomes. As has been argued in studies developing the self-as-doer concept (e.g., Brouwer & Mosack, 2012, 2013; Houser-Marko and Sheldon, 2006), the self-as-doer is different from, albeit related to, constructs that have been used in health behavior change research such as self-determination theory, habit, self-efficacy, locus of control, and outcome expectancies.

As Houser-Marko and Sheldon (2006) have argued, self-determination theory (Deci & Ryan, 1985) is relevant to the self-as-doer construct. Self-determination theory states that people are more likely to persist in behav-iors when they feel intrinsically motivated in doing them (i.e., when they enjoy the very act of the behavior). Furthermore, one may persist in a behav-ior because of "identified motivation" or because a person has identified a desired terminal value for the behavior (e.g., one exercises to be healthy; Deci & Ryan, 1985). The self-as-doer may share some of these attributes, but the self-as-doer also provides explanatory power in cases where behav-iors are not associated with strong terminal values (e.g., checking blood glucose levels only to find out they are in an unacceptable range; Brouwer & Mosack, 2013; Houser-Marko & Sheldon, 2006). The difference between the self-as-doer and self-determination theory is particularly relevant for those engaging in health behaviors that are aversive or difficult and yet desired.

According to self-determination theory, three psychological needs would lead a person to persist in a behavior: autonomy, competence, or related-ness (Deci & Ryan, 1985). That is, a woman with diabetes might follow a diabetes-specific diet because she feels a sense of autonomy and compe-tence when she has completed this task. This sense of reward or satisfaction may reinforce similar behaviors in the future. Yet this claim fails to explain why people may persist in these behaviors when they *do not* express a sense of value or intrinsic motivation. The self-as-doer, on the other hand, can account for persistence even when a sense of autonomy or competence is lacking. As stated by Houser-Marko and Sheldon (2006), "the self-as-doer construct may supply additional explanatory power because it involves identifying with the process of behaving itself as well as with the longer-term values being served by the behavior" (pp. 1037–1038).

It could be argued that if a person who identifies with a doer-behavior is more likely to repeat the behavior in the future, then the simplest explanation for that behavior is that it has become a habit. However, Houser-Marko and Sheldon (2006) reason that the self-as-doer is different from habit because the self-as-doer involves identity and self-schemas which contribute to one's self-concept. Habits are unique in that they prompt automatic behavioral responses due to context cues (Wood & Rünger, 2016). Because habits are automatic responses within a given context, there is no acknowledgement that the self has a role in promoting that behavior. Herein lies how the self-as-doer identity is different; the sense of self is what helps determine behavioral engagement. Those with self-as-doer identities are aware of their behavior as it is part of their self-concept. Therefore, the link between self and behavior is again a distinguishing facet of the self-as-doer theory.

An important concept in self-related theories is self-efficacy. Self-efficacy is the perceived belief in one's ability or capacity to carry out a task or behavior as needed in a particular situation (Scherer, 1982). Taken further, social cognitive theory states that behavior is largely influenced by the belief in one's ability to perform or carry out a specific behavior (Bandura, 1998; Luszczynska & Schwarzer, 2005). Houser-Marko and Sheldon (2006) have posited that the self-as-doer construct is different from self-efficacy because the self-as-doer addresses not just the ability to perform a behavior, but the identification with the *doing* of the behavior. An individual might have the ability to eat fruits, but this may not ultimately determine that the behavior will be carried out. Motivation and persistence are important factors to consider. By linking the sense of self with the action being performed, the self-as-doer provides additional motivational resources beyond levels of ability needed to enact behaviors. Previous research has documented the self-as-doer to be independent of self-efficacy (Brouwer & Feenstra, 2008; Brouwer & Mosack, 2013) when predicting behavior and that self-as-doer identity can explain how self-efficacy affects self-care behaviors in individuals with diabetes (Brouwer & Mosack, 2012).

Another construct of value in the study of health behavior change is the attribution of control. Health behavior interventions have employed elements of control and attribution as per the theory of locus of control (Rotter, 1966). The locus of control theory reflects the extent to which individuals believe that health events, for example, are under their control (internal) or under the control of others (external; see Rotter, 1966; Wallston, Wallston, & DeVellis, 1978; Wallston, Wallston, Kaplan, & Maides, 1976). The self-as-doer construct differs from locus of control in that the self-as-doer is more than just a belief—it is a dynamic agent. Thus, doer-identification may provide further information concerning why individuals may persist in a behavior despite their attribution of control. Regardless of control attribution, individuals pursuing health goals may persist in those behaviors because they see themselves as the doer, an active agent, of their behaviors. Finally, the self-as-doer is different from outcome expectancies. Outcome expectancies are the expectations that a behavior will lead to a desired outcome. While researchers have demonstrated strong relationships between outcome expectancies and behavioral enactment, (Kobau & DiIorio, 2003; Palfai, 2002; Renner, Knoll, & Schwarzer, 2000; Williams, Anderson, & Winett, 2005), the self-as-doer is argued to be a different construct because it is more than just a belief or expectation. Again, because it is an identity in which the self and behavior are linked, it is theorized to be a self-schema of *doing* the behavior, not just an expectation of the behavioral outcome.

Researchers have supported these theoretical distinctions. Houser-Marko and Sheldon (2006) documented that the self-as-doer construct can predict behavior or goal attainment above and beyond goal commitment, self-concordance, expectancies, personality constructs such as openness to experience and neuroticism, and previous experience with goals. Additionally, Brouwer and Mosack (2013) have demonstrated that self-as-doer identity specific to diabetes self-care behaviors can predict engagement in self-care behaviors over and above self-determination, locus of control, illness identity, outcome expectancies, and self-efficacy. Brouwer (n.d.) has also found that the self-as-doer identity specific to physical activity behaviors can predict rates of physical activity after controlling for self-determination, self-efficacy, exercise motivations, and exercise identity. Overall, the self-as-doer has been demonstrated to be theoretically unique and useful in predicting behavior.

Conclusion

The self-as-doer is a novel concept that helps to predict both attractive and aversive behaviors. It is a versatile identity that can be defined broadly or specifically to certain behaviors. As a dynamic agent, the self-as-doer can be activated momentarily or recurrently. It is focused on the self and not on others, and can be "activated" by those who do not already think of themselves as doers. This cognitive representation of the self linked with behavior encourages corresponding behavior and provides a motivational resource. When the self-as-doer is "activated," an individual is more likely to engage in that behavior compared to other similar psychological constructs. Moreover, the unique attributes and ability of the self-as-doer construct to predict behavior have the potential to promote health behavior change and maintenance. The self-as-doer is particularly applicable to health behavior promotion in that it can be activated for both those who do and do not think of themselves as able to engage in health behaviors. Its focus is on *doing* the behavior rather than merely being rewarded by it, and it can be broadly used across multiple health behaviors and in diverse populations. Therefore, the applicability of the self-as-doer to diverse health behaviors in both clinical and non-clinical populations will be the focus of the next chapters.

References

Bandura, A. (1998). Health promotion from the perspective of social cognitive theory. *Psychology and Health, 13,* 623–649. doi: 10.1080/08870449808407422

Brouwer, A. M. (n.d.). *Predicting physical activity with identity: The self-as-doer identity.* Unpublished manuscript.

Brouwer, A. M., & Feenstra, J. S. (2008). *Predictors of self-care behaviors in diabetes: Self-efficacy and self-as-doer.* Unpublished manuscript.

Brouwer, A. M., & Mosack, K. E. (2012). "I am a blood sugar checker": Intervening effects of the self-as-doer identity on the relationship between self-efficacy and diabetes self-care behaviors. *Self and Identity, 11,* 472–491. doi: 10.1080/15298868.2011.603901

Brouwer, A. M., & Mosack, K. E. (2013). Self-as-doer for diabetes: Development and validation of a diabetes-specific measure of doer identification. *Journal of Nursing Measurement, 21,* 188–209. doi: 10.1891/1061–3749.21.2.188

Brouwer, A. M., & Mosack, K. E. (2015). Motivating health diet behaviors: The self-as-doer identity. *Self and Identity, 14,* 638–653. doi: 10.1080/15298868.2015.1043335

Deci, E. L., & Ryan, R. M. (1985). *Intrinsic motivation and self-determination in human behavior.* New York: Plenum Press.

Houser-Marko, L., & Sheldon, K. M. (2006). Motivating behavioral persistence: The self-as-doer construct. *Personality and Social Psychology Bulletin, 32,* 1037–1049. doi: 10.1177/0146167206287974

Kobau, R., & DiIorio, C. (2003). Epilepsy self-management: A comparison of self-efficacy and outcome expectancy for medication adherence and lifestyle behaviors among people with epilepsy. *Epilepsy & Behavior, 4,* 217–225. doi: 10.1016/S1525–5050(03)00057-X

Luszczynska, A., & Schwarzer, R. (2005). Social cognitive theory. In M. Conner, & P. Norman (Eds.), *Predicting health behaviour* (2nd rev. ed., pp. 127–169). Buckingham, England: Open University Press.

Markus, H., & Wurf, E. (1987). The dynamic self-concept: A social psychological perspective. In M. R. Rosenzweig, L. W. Porter, M. R. Rosenzweig, & L. W. Porter (Eds.), *Annual review of psychology* (Vol. 38, pp. 299–337). Palo Alto, CA: Annual Reviews.

Palfai, T. P. (2002). Positive outcome expectancies and smoking behavior: The role of expectancy accessibility. *Cognitive Therapy and Research, 26,* 317–333. doi: 10.1023/A:1016024927094

Renner, B., Knoll, N., & Schwarzer, R. (2000). Age and body make a difference in optimistic health beliefs and nutrition behaviors. *International Journal of Behavioral Medicine, 7,* 143–159. doi: 10.1207/S15327558IJBM0702_4

Rotter, J. B. (1966). Generalized expectancies for internal versus external control of reinforcements. *Psychological Monographs, 80,* 1–28. doi: 10.1037/h0092976

Scherer, M. (1982). The self-efficacy scale: Construction and validation. *Psychological Reports, 15,* 663–671. doi: 10.2466/pr0.1982.51.2.663

Schlenker, B. R., Britt, T. W., Pennington, J., Murphy, R., & Doherty, K. (1994). The triangle model of responsibility. *Psychological Review, 101,* 632–652. doi: 10.1037/0033-295X.101.4.632

Schlenker, B. R., Pontari, B. A., & Christopher, A. N. (2001). Excuses and character: Personal and social implications of excuses. *Personality and Social Psychology Review, 5,* 15–32. doi: 10.1207/S15327957PSPR0501_2

Stets, J. E., & Burke, P. J. (2000). Identity theory and social identity theory. *Social Psychology Quarterly, 63,* 224–237. doi: 10.2307/2695870

Strachan, S. M., & Brawley, L. R. (2008). Reactions to a perceived challenge to identity: A focus on exercise and healthy eating. *Journal of Health Psychology, 13,* 575–588. doi: 10.1177/1359105308090930

Strachan, S. M., & Brawley, L. R. (2009). Healthy-eater identity and self-efficacy predict healthy eating behavior: A prospective view. *Journal of Health Psychology, 14,* 684–695. doi: 10.1177/1359105309104915

Wallston, B. S., Wallston, K. A., Kaplan, G. D., & Maides, S. A. (1976). Development of the health locus of control (HLC) scale. *Journal of Consulting Clinical Psychology, 44,* 580–585. doi: 10.1037/0022-006X.44.4.580

Wallston, K. A., Wallston, B. S., & DeVellis, R. (1978). Development of the multidimensional health locus of control (MHLC) scales. *Health Education Monograph, 6,* 160–170. doi: 10.1177/109019817800600107

Walsh, R. S., Muldoon, O. T., Gallagher, S., & Fortune, D. G. (2015). Affiliative and "self-as-doer" identities: Relationship between social identity, social support and emotional status amongst survivors of acquired brain injury (ABI). *Neuropsychological Rehabilitation, 25,* 555–573. doi: 10.1080/09602011.2014.993658

Williams, D. M., Anderson, E. S., & Winett, R. A. (2005). A review of the outcome expectancies in physical activity research. *Annals of Behavioral Medicine, 29,* 70–79. doi: 10.1207/s15324796abm2901_10

Wood, W., & Rünger, D. (2016). Psychology of habit. *Annual Review of Psychology, 67,* 289–314. doi: 10.1146/annurev-psych-122414-033417

3 Creating Self-as-Doer Identities

The theoretical nature of the self-as-doer identity is such that a self-concept is linked with behavior. What makes the self-as-doer unique is that it is an identity describing the active agent, *the doer*, of a behavior. In creating self-as-doer identities, the active agent is operationalized by adding an -er suffix to the action of a goal phrase. Consider, for example, that an individual has the goal of eating healthy. The action, the verb, of the phrase is to "eat." Adding an -er suffix to the verb then transforms the action of "eating" to being an "eater." The object in the goal phrase is then used to specify what sort of active agent the individual is conceptualizing. In the case of "eating healthy," the object is "healthy." Putting the newly constructed verb together with the object, the goal of "eating healthy" is then transformed into a doer of healthy eating—a "healthy eater" (Brouwer & Mosack, 2015). The idea behind creating self-as-doer identities is that the individual is able to change his or her goal into a statement that describes the individual doing the goal. Thus the goal to "walk daily" becomes "daily walker," the goal of taking medication becomes "medication taker," and the goal of "going to the gym" becomes "gym go-er." It is important to note that not all doer identities follow grammatical conventions. Examples from research include "sugar cutter backer," "home cooker," and "yoga doer" (Brouwer, n.d.; Brouwer & Mosack, 2015). Yet, the doer identities are developed from self-determined goals which provide a unique sense of meaning for the individual who created them and, consequently, a connection with the identity that is likely to elicit motivation for behavior in accordance with the identity.

How descriptive the doer identities are is left up to the individual creating them. In the aforementioned examples of doer identities (e.g., "daily walker"), only the object and verb are used. However, the author can create more specific doer phrases depending upon his or her specific goals. For example, if the frequency of the goal is particularly important, then a frequency modifier could also be included in the development of the doer identity. For instance, if an individual has a goal of "eating vegetables daily," the verb of the goal phrase is to "eat" and the object is "vegetables." One could create a simple doer identity of "vegetable eater," but if the behavior of eating vegetables on a daily basis is a fundamental part of the goal, then this too should be included in the creation of the doer identity. That is, the adverb indicating the frequency of the behavior could also be used in the doer phrase. So rather than only a "vegetable eater," the doer identity would be "daily vegetable eater."

The motivational orientation of doer identities can be either approach- or avoidant-oriented. Elliot (2006) defines approach motivation as the orientation of a behavior in a positive direction, moving toward positive stimuli (e.g., run 3 times a week), whereas avoidance motivation is moving away from negative stimuli (e.g., abstain from watching TV). Since the doer identity is created from goals, doer identities can embrace either orientation (e.g., "high-fat food avoider" or "low-fat food eater"). Individuals do, however, tend to create more approach-oriented doer phrases than avoidant-oriented ones (Brouwer & Mosack, 2013, 2015). Another important facet of creating doer identities is that each identity needs to describe the individual doing the goal as the active agent. It cannot simply be an identity; it must link the self with the behavior. If an individual was considering lifting weights more intensely and created a goal of "to lift weights like a warrior," an identity as a "weight lifting warrior" would not reflect the theoretical nature of the self-as-doer identity because it does not link the identity with the behavior; a warrior is not a behavior. "Weight lifting warrior" only describes the identity. The correct doer phrase, in this example, would be "warrior weight lifter" because here the behavior of lifting weights is now linked with the identity of a warrior.

In the process of creating doer identities, it is important that the individual creating them has the flexibility to make each phrase personally meaningful. Research demonstrates that self-determined goals, especially those related to health behaviors, are more effective in achieving desired outcomes than those that are prescribed or assigned (Estabrooks et al., 2005; Pearson, 2012; Ryan & Deci, 2000). For example, a woman may have a goal related to losing weight and therefore could create a doer identity as "weight loser," but if she conceptualizes the goal as "to wear size 8 jeans," then a doer identity as a "size 8 jean wearer" might be more relevant and motivating for her. Although a doer identity as "size 8 jean wearer" may feel too distant from the behaviors of losing weight or may even elicit some degree of laughter in the process of developing serious health goals, it is meaningful for the individual. Moreover, the doer identity of a "size 8 jean wearer" likely includes behaviors that are appropriate for healthy weight maintenance (e.g., exercising regularly, eating a healthy diet) thereby making the identity relevant to behaviors required for weight loss. As such, this personal identity, the engendered self-concept linked with behavior, can be a source of motivation and persistence for this individual because it is personalized.

Measuring Self-as-Doer Identity

Measuring self-as-doer identity requires a multi-step process aimed at linking a self-concept with behavior and evaluating the degree to which one can identify with this new doer identity. The steps for this process include (1) creating goals, (2) transforming goals into doer identities, and (3) rating the degree to which each of the doer identities describes the self.

Step 1: Creating Goals

In the first step, participants identify and list three to eight goals that are either general (e.g., inclusive of several goals from diverse behaviors) or domain-specific (e.g., physical activity goals). In research establishing the construct, Houser-Marko and Sheldon (2006) asked participants to list eight general goals. Participants could list diverse goals from any realm of their lives (e.g., academic, social, etc.) to represent an overall, general doer identity score. This doer identity represented the ability to see oneself as a doer across multiple behaviors. Upon finding low reliability in the measure, the researchers modified the measure in a subsequent study and asked participants to create three goals (instead of eight) that were specific to one particular behavior (i.e., domain-specific goals). Having fewer goals that were specific to a behavior resulted in better reliability of the measure. In other research exploring diet, physical activity, and self-care behaviors for individuals with diabetes, participants were asked to identify six goals (Brouwer, n.d.; Brouwer & Mosack, 2012, 2013, 2015). The measure was found to have adequate reliability with six goals in domain-specific areas of research, as well. How the self-as-doer is measured, whether it is general or domain-specific, is determined by researchers' interests and, consequently, the instructions given to those completing the measure. Both forms have had success in measuring self-as-doer identity; however, individuals who create goals that are more specific tend to have better success in enacting corresponding behavior change (Pearson, 2012; Strecher et al., 1995).

Step 2: Creating Doer Identities

After completing the goal statements, participants are then instructed on how to create doer identities from each goal. A sample of the instructions from a diet study (Brouwer & Mosack, 2015) that was modified from Houser-Marko and Sheldon's (2006) study are as follows:

> Every personal goal contains both a *verb* and an *object*. For example, for the goal "to eat more fruits" the verb is *eat* and the object is *fruits*. For the goal "to consume less salt" the verb is *consume less* and the object is *salt*. I would like you to think about the verb and object in each of the healthy eating goals you have and create a *special phrase* using the "er" suffix. Place this in the second blank above next to each goal statement (1b, 2b, 3b, etc.). This phrase will refer to a *person who does the goal*. For example, the goal "to eat more fruits" might be rephrased "fruit eater." The goal "to consume less salt" might be rephrased "less salt consumer."

Participants then create a doer phrase for each of their goal statements. Interventionists and researchers should assist participants as needed. Although it is possible to complete the self-as-doer measure without assistance, the reliability and validity of the measure is bolstered when participants can get immediate correction on doer identities that are created incorrectly. That is, if a phrase is not created with an -er suffix the researcher can offer a suggestion to frame the doer identity in this way; or if the transformed verb does not reflect an active behavioral response (e.g., "haver" or "be-er"), the interventionist or researcher can assist the participant in choosing a more appropriate verb phrase. Likewise, if the participant needs suggestions for getting started, the researcher can offer an example of how to modify a goal to create a doer identity phrase.

Step 3: Rating Doer Identities

In the final step, participants rate on a scale of 1 (does not describe me well) to 5 (describes me very well) the degree to which the doer identity describes them. The act of conceptualizing the doer phrase (e.g., imagining what a "healthy eater" does and looks like, and then determining the level to which the phrase describes oneself) is an important process in evaluating one's doer identity. The cognitive processes undertaken when defining the behaviors of a doer and then relating these attributes back to oneself are unique processes differing from the steps of creating goals and developing special doer phrases. After a rating has been assigned to each doer identity, the aggregated doer identity is then computed by finding the average score from doer identity ratings. An example of the self-as-doer measure as was used in Brouwer and Mosack (2015), is as follows:

Self-as-Doer Measure

Now that you have read about healthy eating, we would like you to complete this task. For the survey below I would like you to think about 6 goals related to healthy eating. Please write them on the first line/or in the space after each number (1, 2, 3, 4). Leave the second line/space (1b, 2b, etc.) blank until further instructions.

1. _____   1b. _____

2. _____   2b. _____

3. _____   3b. _____

4. _____   4b. _____

5. _____   5b. _____

6. _____   6b. _____

Further instructions

Every personal goal contains both a *verb* and an *object*.

> For example, for the goal "to eat more fruits" the verb is *eat* and the object is *fruits*.
> For the goal "to consume less salt" the verb is *consume less* and the object is *salt*.

I would like you to think about the verb and object in each of the healthy eating goals you have and create a *special phrase* using the "er" suffix. Place this in the second blank above (1b, 2b, 3b, etc.).
This phrase will refer to a *person who does the goal.*

> For example, the goal "to eat more fruits" might be rephrased "fruit eater."
> The goal "to consume less salt" might be rephrased "less salt consumer."

Complete this task and then read the rest of these directions (example statements can be used).

Now that you have written down your goals and the special phrase please indicate how well the special phrase describes or fits you using the scale given below. Please put the number on the line/space in front of each number below corresponding to the above numbers.

How well does the 'er' phrase describe you?

Does Not Describe Me Well At All	Does Not Describe Me Well	Neutral	Describes Me Well	Describes Me Very Well
1	2	3	4	5

_____ 1.   _____ 3.   _____ 5.

_____ 2.   _____ 4.   _____ 6.

Examples of Self-as-Doer Identities
From Health Behavior Research

To better understand how doer identities take form in the context of health behaviors, three studies where doer identities were created related to diet, physical activity, and diabetes-specific self-care behaviors will be reviewed. More specifically, the content of doer phrases for each study will be discussed, and examples of commonly used doer phrases will be provided as examples of how the self-as-doer task takes shape in health-related contexts.

Diet Behaviors

In a study exploring the how doer identity can influence healthy eating behaviors, participants were asked to construct six goals related to healthy eating (Brouwer & Mosack, 2015). As part of the experimental condition, participants reviewed general nutrition education materials created by the United States Department of Agriculture (USDA) before creating doer identities (USDA, 2010a, 2010b, 2010c). Nutrition guidelines provided recommendations such as building a healthy plate which included making the half the plate fruits and vegetables, switching to skim or 1% milk, making half of grains eaten in a day whole grains, and eating more seafood or natural sources of fiber and protein. Cutting back on high-fat foods and foods with added sugar and salt, eating the right amount of calories, and suggested ways to get more physically active were also recommended in the USDA materials. In addition to the general guidelines, participants also read tip sheets for making these recommendations applicable. Some tips included trying new foods, using a smaller plate, taking time to eat food, drinking more water, and eating at home more often. Although the educational materials served both as a primer and resource for creating appropriate healthy eating goals, participants were allowed to create any goals (and subsequent doer identities) related to healthy eating.

In the first step, participants created goals related to healthy eating behaviors. From a content analysis, these goals primarily reflected eating more fruits and vegetables. Example goals included, "Eat more fruit," "Eat 4 servings of veggies a day," and "Grab the veggie tray vs. crackers." Participants also created goals for eating more whole grains (e.g., "Eat whole grain pasta"), low-fat dairy products (e.g., "Try 1% milk"), lean meats (e.g., "Eat leaner protein"), drinking more water (e.g., "Drink more water"), and reducing sugar-sweetened beverages (e.g., "Drink less soda"). Some goals reflected modifying the techniques of eating, including a focus on portion control (e.g., "Use a smaller plate," "Make sure to eat slower," "Make smaller portions," "Cook at home more often"), restricting certain food groups (e.g., "Eat fewer foods with solid fats," "Consume less sodium"), and managing caloric intake (e.g., "Balance calories"). In the second step, participants created doer identities. In a content analysis of the created doer identity phrases, the majority of participants created self-as-doer identities related to vegetable ($n = 23$; 92%) and fruit ($n = 22$; 88%) consumption. Many created identities that described the direct behavior of eating more fruits and vegetables by creating phrases such as, "veggie eater," "fruit eater," and "more veggies consumer." Some even described what kinds of fruits and vegetables to eat through phrases such as "wide variety of fruits eater," "dark green vegetable eater," "warm or cooked veggie eater," and "colorful veggie eater." Others created doer identities that described how to eat more fruits and vegetables by fitting more fruits and vegetables into one's diet (e.g., "more vegetable fitter inner," "fruit includer," and "extra fruit eater"), and exchanging fruit for existing foods in one's diet (e.g., "fresh fruit swapper" and "fruit for dessert eater"). Some doer identities also explicitly mirrored recommendations provided by the USDA in the educational materials presented in the study. Example phrases included, "1/2 plate fruit and veggie eater" and "2–3 serving vegetable eater."

Approximately 40% ($n = 10$) of participants created doer identities related to whole grains (e.g., "whole grain eater," "whole grains adder," "whole grains product eater"), 36% ($n = 9$) created identities for low-fat dairy or adding calcium to one's diet (e.g., "calcium eater/drinker," "skim milk drinker"), and 24% ($n = 6$) of participants created identities related to reducing sugar-sweetened beverages. Since the USDA recommendations for healthy eating are to restrict or reduce sugar-sweetened beverages, many of the doer identities created for this behavior were avoidant orientated (e.g., "less soda drinker," "less sugary drink drinker").

Other doer identities commonly created were identities representing goals for particular techniques for eating behaviors ($n = 23$; 92%); that is, behaviors for how food was eaten or in what forms. For example, participants created identities such as "small plate user," "slower eater," "scheduled eater," "non-late night snacker," "family eater," and "homemade meal maker." Another category included identities endorsing some form of restrictive eating such as cutting back or eating less of non-healthy food items ($n = 16$; 64%). These included identities such as "less sodium consumer," "sugar reducer," "less fried food eater," "carbohydrate limiter," "oversized portion avoider," and "fat cutter backer." The remainder of doer identities included identities related to eating more lean meats (e.g., "leaner proteins eater," "fish eater," "seafood eater"); controlling portion sizes (e.g., "smaller portion eater," "small plate/bowl user," and "smaller meat portion eater"); drinking more water (e.g., "more water drinker"); adhering to specific diet plans (e.g., "actually hungry eater," "appropriate calorie eater," "satisfied eater," "healthy sweet tooth satisfier"); trying new foods (e.g., "new foods trier," "new foods explorer"); incorporating more fiber (e.g., "fiber eater"); and using different cooking techniques (e.g., "different oil user," "creative home meal preparer"). Only 5 of the 150 created doer identities were not specific to food. However, these identities did represent healthy behaviors such as physical activity (e.g., "physical runner/walker"), getting adequate sleep (e.g., "sleeper"), losing weight (e.g., "weight maintainer," "weight loser"), and having healthy skin (e.g., "healthy skin getter").

In sum, self-as-doer identities can be successfully used within a diet framework. Given the prompts for healthy eating, researchers were able to elicit doer identities that were in line with the objectives of the study. Participants created diverse identities reflecting not just eating behaviors but also environmental conditions to help support those behaviors (e.g., "small plate user," "home cooker"). Furthermore, the breadth of doer phrases was large, thereby suggesting that this task can include the many relevant diet-related doer identities that individuals may have in their healthy eating behaviors.

Physical Activity Behaviors

In a study exploring how self-as-doer identity is related to physical activity, 220 participants were asked to create doer identities specific to physical activity behaviors (Brouwer, n.d.). Prior to developing the doer identities, participants reviewed general physical activity recommendations in a booklet published by the Department of Health and Human Services (DHHS; DHHS, 2008). In the booklet, participants first reviewed different types of activities (e.g., aerobic, strengthening) and the DHHS's recommendations for the amount of physical activity needed each week relative to the different types of activities (e.g., 2 hours and 30 minutes of aerobic activity that requires moderate effort). Several examples of moderate and vigorous activities and tips for maintenance were provided (e.g., having a support network, finding time that works best, mixing up one's activities to avoid boredom). Participants also reviewed specific recommendations relative to their existing physical activity routines. For example, if a participant was not currently physically active or had a very low rate of physical activity, there was a designated section of the booklet that outlined how to get started with physical activity and included tips such as starting slow and building up over time and choosing activities that fit into one's life. Other sections for those who were already somewhat active identified ways to add more activity to existing routines with recommendations such as going longer, being active on more days a week, choosing activities that work more parts of the body, and adding more effort to existing workouts (i.e., changing from moderate to vigorous activities). The benefits of physical activity, ways to avoid injury, and methods for tracking physical activity were also described in the booklet.

In analyzing the first step of doer identity creation, we found that participants created goals which reflected diverse forms of physical activity. Example goals statements include, "run 5 days a week," "start Pilates," "do more biking," "become more flexible," "play cricket," and "canoe once a week when possible." Participants also created goals that identified the degree of intensity or frequency of their physical activity behaviors (e.g., "do yoga 2–3 times a week," "run for a longer duration on treadmill," "do moderate activities twice a week"). Others identified barriers to their physical activity behaviors (e.g., "find the time (to workout)"), and some developed goals that reflected ways to overcome some of the barriers (e.g., "take stairs more often," "park farther from campus," "wake up earlier," "instead of TV, bike ride").

The results of a content analysis of doer identities indicated that participants created diverse identities not just related to engaging in specific physical activity behaviors, but also identities related to the environment needed to ensure the success of carrying out the related behaviors. Of the 1,316 doer identities created, 598 (45%) were identities that described performing behaviors. Sample statements include, "weight lifter," "rollerblader," "racquet baller," "jogger," "Zumba-er," "gym goer," and "stairs taker." Within this category there were identities that specifically reflected joining a class or participating in a structured event (e.g., "fitness class joiner," "intermural joiner," "butt-n-gut (class) go-er"). When creating identities for this category, some participants also included the frequency in which the behaviors would be performed (e.g., "once a week yoga class go-er," "3x a week lifter," "4 day exerciser," "every day runner"). In addition to creating doer identities focused on behavior, participants also created identities describing the intensity of behaviors in general (e.g., "moderate activity participator," "higher vigorous activity doer," "vigorous cardio doer"). It is likely that these identities, in particular, may have been primed by the DHHS recommendations. In the same way that doer identities related to diet invoked context, many of the doer identities related to physical activity also considered the environment in which one would enact the doer identity.

Participants also created doer identities specific to new behaviors (e.g., "new workout trier," "beginning runner," "exercise starter") and modifying existing physical activity routines. Identities that focused on modifying existing routines often reflected increasing activities (e.g., "endurance level increaser," "exercise time increaser," "farther and longer walker"), and improving performance (e.g., "stamina improver," "agility improver"). In several of the doer identities ($n = 68$; 5%), participants described ways that would assist them in making physical activity changes. For example, some described how they would increase physical activity while engaging in other sedentary behaviors. One participant noted that she would try to move more while studying and consequently created a doer identity as "moving studier." Others created identities for moving while watching television shows or movies (e.g., "Netflix walker").

Participants also created identities for behaviors that would require them to engage in physical activity in order to achieve another goal like getting somewhere (e.g., "further parker," "taker of the long path," "biker instead of driver"). Others created identities that described behaviors necessary for incorporating physical activity into their lives (e.g., "goal setter," "priority maker," "habit builder," "progress tracker"). Finally, several participants created identities that would remove barriers for engaging in physical activity (e.g., "non-social media user," "minimal TV watcher," "earlier riser").

In addition to creating identities that would describe behaviors or ways to engage in those behaviors, participants also created identities reflecting the need to include others in their behaviors (e.g., "partner workout-er," "friend canoer," "social walker"). Some doer identities, although very few, also reflected non-specific behaviors related to overall health (e.g., "health maintainer," "physical activity doer"). Finally, there was a category of doer identities ($n = 173$; 13%) that described health behaviors that were not specific to physical activity. Many of these were diet-related (e.g., "healthy eater," "organic food eater," "water drinker") and some described sleep- (e.g., "earlier sleeper") and weight-related (e.g., "weight loser") behaviors.

In regards to the type of physical activity behaviors participants created goals and doer identities for, participants created identities with a broad range of behaviors. Doer identities phrases were related to flexibility (e.g., "stretcher"), strength training (e.g., "weight lifter"), cardiovascular training (e.g., "runner"), and everyday activities (e.g., "stair taker," "stander"). Doer identities also represented both individual (e.g., "runner") and team sport (e.g., "volleyball player") activities.

As with doer identities related to diet, doer identities for physical activity can be successfully created in a way that can be used to promote health behavior change and maintenance. Doer identities reflected diverse physical activities from a broad scope of behaviors, with many including frequencies of the behavior, adding or modifying existing behaviors, and establishing ways to create an environment supportive of engaging in physical activity.

Diabetes-Specific Self-Care Behaviors

Diabetes requires consistent self-care management and adherence to a set of prescribed self-care behaviors (e.g., healthy eating, being active, monitoring, taking medication, problem solving, risk reduction, and healthy coping;

American Diabetes Association [ADA], 2016; Shirvastava, Shrivastava, & Ramasamy, 2013). As such, having an identity as a doer of one's self-care behaviors, particularly for behaviors that are not necessarily reinforcing or rewarding, may provide additional motivation to engage in and sustain self-care behaviors. Therefore, Brouwer (2008) conducted a study to determine whether the self-as-doer identity could predict diabetes self-care behaviors. Goals and doer identities from 92 individuals with diabetes were analyzed for content. Many participants created goals related to healthy eating (e.g., "follow a low-fat diet," "count calories more efficiently," "eat healthier") with the majority of food-related goals reflecting limiting or restricting certain foods (e.g., "try to resist sweets," "limit high-fat treats," "resist unhealthy foods"). Participants also created goals that reflected blood glucose management (e.g., "tighter blood sugar control," "be more aware of my highs and lows," "get my sugars more tightly controlled") and achieving a good hemoglobin A1c (e.g., "get my A1c under 7," "maintain good A1c"). Goal statements also reflected self-care management behaviors related to exercise (e.g., "exercise more," "continue to exercise regularly"), blood glucose monitoring (e.g., "test blood sugars daily"), weight management (e.g., "loose and keep off 15 pounds"), foot care (e.g., "check my feet weekly") and relationships with health care professionals (e.g., "see my doctor more regularly," "follow doctor's advice").

Results of the content analysis for doer identities demonstrated that the majority of doer identities reflected the ADA guidelines for self-care behavior. Out of 452 doer identities created, approximately 22% (*n* = 100) were associated with diet. The most popular category of doer identity related to diet was associated with resisting or limiting certain foods in their diet (e.g., "sweets resister," "high-fat limiter," "limited snacker," "dessert avoider"). Other identities related to diet regimen focused on carbohydrate counting (e.g., "accurate carb counter," "less carb eater"). Although a few doer identities were specific to eating certain types of foods (e.g., "more fruit and veggie eater"), most phrases were broad, with identities focused on having a better diet or a more healthier diet in general (e.g., "better eater," "healthy food eater," "healthier eater," "diet follower").

The next most common category of doer identities was related to hemoglobin A1c and blood glucose levels (19%, *n* = 86). Hemoglobin A1c is a measure of the average glucose in the blood over a 3–4 month period and is often used by medical professionals as a measure of adherence and diabetes health (ADA, 2016). Many doer identities within this category reflected the goals of achieving adequate A1c levels (e.g., "good A1c getter," "good A1c maintainer," "better A1c getter"). Although the majority of doer identities created reflected a general level of achievement (good, better, etc.), some doer identities reflected specific goals. For example, some identities included "under 7 A1c keeper" and "A1c below 7.1 getter." Other identities within this category described behaviors related to blood glucose control. Example identities include, "tight sugar controller," "good blood sugar controller," "better blood sugar controller," and "hyperglycemia avoider."

Participants also created phrases related to physical activity levels (17%, $n = 76$). Although some were specific to certain activities (e.g., "frequent gym goer," "successful runner"), the majority of identities were general and often included of the desired frequency of physical activity engagement (e.g., "daily exerciser," "regular exerciser," "habitual exerciser"). Doer identities related to blood glucose monitoring (10%, $n = 44$) were also created and like physical activity, they reflected general behaviors (e.g., "frequent blood sugar tester," "regular blood sugar tester") and monitoring tied to a specific event (e.g., "meal time tester," "nighttime sugar tester"). Also in line with the ADA recommendations for diabetes self-care, several participants created doer identities related to medication or insulin adherence (4%, $n = 16$). These identities primarily described taking medication (e.g., "good insulin taker," "bolus taker") or engaging in a modification of the current regimen (e.g., "medication/insulin reducer," "more aggressive insulin giver," "better medication timer"). In addition to the primary self-care behavior recommendations from the ADA, doer identities (9%, $n = 41$) also reflected several secondary care behaviors such as eye care (e.g., "eye exam getter," "eye complications avoider") and foot care (e.g., "frequent food checker," "good foot examiner").

Outside of more traditional recommendations for diabetes self-care behavior management, participants created doer identities specific to improving their knowledge about diabetes ("diabetes educator," "diabetes knower"; 1%, $n = 6$); use of technology ("insulin pump getter," "better basal rate adjuster," "site changer"; 6%, $n = 30$); record keeping skills (e.g., "regular logger," "good documenter"; 1%, $n = 6$); and timeliness in medical appointment making (e.g., "attentive appointment holder"; 0.4%, $n = 2$). Participants also focused on enhancing their relationships with their team of health care professionals ("regular doctor examiner," "good communicator"; 2%; $n = 10$) and giving and receiving social support ("support group attender," "diabetes event participator"; 2%, $n = 11$). Participants also created doer identities related to financial responsibilities ("financial helper"; 0.4%, $n = 2$) and research participation ("researcher," "supporter"; 1%, $n = 8$).

Finally, participants created doer identities (15%, $n = 69$) that reflected more general health behaviors including weight management (e.g., "weight maintainer," "weight loser"); getting adequate sleep (e.g., "good sleeper," "cloud 9 dreamer"); quitting smoking (e.g., "non-smoker," "smoking quitter"); taking vitamins (e.g., "vitamins taker); coping with and managing stress (e.g., "stress handler," "life balancer"); and general overall health (e.g., "good caretaker," "happy and healthy liver").

In addition to general health behaviors like diet and physical activity, the self-as-doer identity can also be specifically targeted to reflect behaviors for chronic illness management. The doer identities that participants created generally mirrored guidelines that medical professionals and the ADA recommend. The vast majority of those created represented the core behaviors for diabetes management (e.g., diet, blood glucose monitoring, physical activity, medication). However, unlike the doer identities created by non-clinical populations for diet and physical activity, individuals with diabetes created more general identities for behavior (e.g., "regular exerciser," "healthy diet eater") versus those with a specific context as was created in the other studies (e.g., "fruit eater," "2x a week runner"). Perhaps the complexity of disease care management prevented individuals from creating specific diet and physical activity goals as did those in the other studies. Nonetheless, results support the versatile nature of using the self-as-doer identity in health behavior promotion and maintenance; the self-as-doer identity can be successfully applied to both general heath behaviors and specifically for disease management behaviors.

Conclusion

Throughout this chapter, the self-as-doer identity has been described as a construct that links the self with behavior. Measurement of this identity reflects the process of developing a cognitive representation of a doer of the behavior and evaluating the degree to which one can describe oneself as the doer of that behavior. The self-as-doer is flexible but can be targeted to reflect recommendations for a variety of health behaviors including healthy eating, physical activity, and management of a chronic illness. Examples from diet and physical activity behaviors suggest that doer identities can take diverse forms within each of these behaviors and describe not only the behavior of eating or exercising, but also identities that help form an environment to support those behaviors. Furthermore, the creation of doer identities specific to a population with a chronic illness demonstrate that doer identities can also reflect disease-specific management that follows traditional and non-traditional regimens. That the self-as-doer is versatile supports its use in health promotion. Given the research that suggests that with some priming doer identities can be created for both general and specific health behaviors, the self-as-doer identity has potential to be used within a wide array of health behaviors for both clinical and non-clinical populations. What follows in the next few chapters is research demonstrating just this—that self-as-doer identities can predict and change health behaviors in both clinical and non-clinical populations.

References

American Diabetes Association (2016). Standards of medical care in diabetes—2016. *Diabetes Care, 39*(1, Suppl), S1–S12.

Brouwer, A. M. (2008, May). *Predictors of self-care behaviors: Self-efficacy and self-as-doer*. Poster presented at the Midwestern Psychological Association Conference in Chicago, IL.

Brouwer, A. M. (n.d.). *Predicting physical activity with identity: The self-as-doer identity*. Unpublished manuscript.

Brouwer, A. M., & Mosack, K. E. (2012). "I am a blood sugar checker": Intervening effects of the self-as-doer identity on the relationship between self-efficacy and diabetes self-care behaviors. *Self and Identity, 11*, 472–491. doi: 10.1080/15298868.2011.603901

Brouwer, A. M., & Mosack, K. E. (2013). Self-as-doer for diabetes: Development and validation of a diabetes-specific measure of doer identification. *Journal of Nursing Measurement, 21*, 188–209. doi: 10.1891/1061-3749.21.2.188

Brouwer, A. M., & Mosack, K. E. (2015). Motivating health diet behaviors: The self-as-doer identity. *Self and Identity, 14*, 638–653. doi: 10.1080/15298868.2015.1043335

Department of Health and Human Services (2008). *2008 physical activity guidelines for Americans*. Retrieved from https://health.gov/paguidelines/pdf/paguide.pdf

Elliot, A. J. (2006). The hierarchical model of approach-avoidance motivation. *Motivation and Emotion, 30*, 111–116. doi: 10.1007/s11031-006-9028-7

Estabrooks, P. A., Nelson, C. C., Xu, S., King, D., Bayliss, E. A., Gaglio, B., . . . Glasgow, R. E. (2005). The frequency and behavioral outcomes of goal choices in the self-management of diabetes. *The Diabetes Educator, 31*, 391–400. doi: 10.1177/0145721705276578

Houser-Marko, L., & Sheldon, K. M. (2006). Motivating behavioral persistence: The self-as-doer construct. *Personality and Social Psychology Bulletin, 32*, 1037–1049. doi: 10.1177/0146167206287974

Pearson, E. S. (2012). Goal setting as a health behavior change strategy in overweight and obese adults: A systematic literature review examining intervention components. *Patient Education and Counseling, 87*(1), 32–42. doi: 10.1016/j.pec.2011.07.018

Ryan, R. M., & Deci, E. L. (2000). Self-determination theory and the facilitation of intrinsic motivation, social development, and well-being. *American Psychologist, 55*(1), 68–78. doi: 10.1037/0003–066X.55.1.68

Shirvastava, S. R., Shrivastava, P. S., & Ramasamy, J. (2013). Role of self-care in management of diabetes mellitus. *Journal of Diabetes & Metabolic Disorders, 12*, 1–5. doi: 10.1186/2251-6581-12-14

Strecher, V. J., Seijts, G. H., Kok, G. J., Latham, G. P., Glasgow, R., DeVellis, B., . . . Bulger, D. W. (1995). Goal setting as a strategy for health behavior change. *Health Education Quarterly, 22*(2), 190–200. doi: 10.1177/109019819502200207

U.S. Department of Agriculture (2010a). *Let's eat for the health of it.* Retrieved from www.choosemyplate.gov/sites/default/files/audiences/DG2010Brochure.pdf

U.S. Department of Agriculture (2010b). *Build a healthy meal.* Retrieved from www.choosemyplate.gov/sites/default/files/tentips/DGTipsheet38BuildHealthy MealtimeHabits_0.pdf

U.S. Department of Agriculture (2010c). *Choose MyPlate 10 tips to a great plate.* Retrieved from www.choosemyplate.gov/sites/default/files/tentips/DGTipsheet1 ChooseMyPlate.pdf

4 Self-as-Doer Identity and Health Behavior Change Within Non-Clinical Populations

Adopting and maintaining healthy lifestyle behaviors is key to acquiring optimal health (Loef & Walach, 2012; Nicklett et al., 2012; Riekert, Ockene, & Pbert, 2014; Thorpe et al., 2013). Researchers have identified several health behaviors (e.g., getting regular physical activity, eating a healthy diet, smoking cessation, and limited alcohol consumption) that contribute to better health and the reduction of disease risk (Ford, Zhao, Tsai, & Li, 2011; Riekert et al., 2014). Moreover, researchers have found that engaging in a combination of these health behaviors has the potential to reduce mortality risks by 66% (Loef & Walach, 2012). Although the importance of engaging in a variety of healthy lifestyle behaviors is well documented, few individuals successfully engage in needed health behavior changes and of those that do, sustaining that change proves difficult. For example, those who enroll in weight loss programs are often successful in the short term, but then gain the lost weight back within 3–5 years (Avenell et al., 2004; Dombrowski, Knittle, Avenell, Araujo-Soares, & Sniehotta, 2014; Foster et al., 2010). Smoking cessation programs have similar results with many individuals relapsing within 6 months (Agboola, Mcneill, Coleman, & Leonardi, 2010; Jones, Lewis, Parrot, Wormall, & Coleman, 2016). Physical activity and diet interventions have been found to have some promise with behavior change, but are still limited in the degree to which that change is maintained overtime, especially for physical activity (Fjeldsoe, Neuhaus, Winkler, & Eakin, 2011; Kroeze, Werkman, & Brug, 2006). Given that 40% of premature deaths can be accounted for by suboptimal health behaviors (Spruijt-Metz et al., 2015), finding ways to motivate change and maintenance of that change are vital for achieving good health. As has been argued thus far, the self-as-doer identity is likely to be a useful factor in not only creating behavioral change for healthy lifestyle behaviors but also promoting the maintenance of that change. To better understand the how the self-as-doer influences health behaviors and how it can be used within non-clinical populations, the relevant outcomes from two studies, one on physical activity and one with diet, will be discussed.

Self-as-Doer Identity and Physical Activity Behaviors (The Physical Activity Study)

Being physically active on a regular basis is important for achieving optimal health. Individuals who are regularly active benefit from reduced risk of various diseases, improved mood, and generally enjoy a longer life expectancy (Center for Disease Control, 2015). However, as with many healthy lifestyle behaviors, there are several barriers (e.g., lack of time and motivation, monetary costs, fatigue, lack of social support, etc.) that prevent individuals from making and sustaining the behavior change needed to reduce risk and improve health (Barnidge et al., 2013; Joseph, Ainsworth, Keller, & Dodgson, 2015; Macniven et al., 2014; Martins, Marques, Sarmento, & da Costa, 2015). Likewise, motivation for behavior change may be low and, consequently, individuals lack the needed impetus to continue efforts at behavior change.

Given that a self-as-doer identity provides motivation to engage in behaviors, particularly when they are not reinforcing, Brouwer (n.d.) conducted a cross-sectional study to determine the role that self-as-doer identity has in overcoming barriers for physical activity and how doer identity is related to existing motivational constructs that affect physical activity behaviors. In this study, participants completed questions assessing their motivations for exercise, exercise identity, self-efficacy for exercise behaviors, and self-efficacy for overcoming barriers to exercising. Participants also reviewed educational materials about physical activity behaviors (i.e., the *Physical Activity Guidelines for Americans* published by the Department of Health and Human Services, 2008) and completed the self-as-doer measure (see Chapter 3 in this volume for an overview of this protocol). For the self-as-doer measure, participants were asked to develop six physical activity-specific goals and to then transform those goals into doer identities. Priming participants with the *Physical Activity Guidelines for Americans* was important for their creation of goals and doer identities in that it provided a resource for knowing what good and recommended physical activity behaviors look like. Moreover, it gave many examples of physical activities that could be specified to each individual's current levels of physical activity. Although the introduction of this material may have affected the creation of doer phrases in that many of the phrases corresponded perfectly with the recommendations (see Chapter 3 in this volume for examples of doer identities), the benefits of the educational primer, particularly that participants would have goals that adequately and appropriately reflected the target behavior, outweighed these disadvantages and served to assist participants in creating doer identities that could be used to motivate and sustain the type of physical activity that would lead to health benefits and disease risk reduction. After creating doer identities, participants then rated each doer identity on a 1 ("does not describe me well at all") to 5 ("describes me very well") scale for the degree to which the identity currently described them. Participants created diverse doer identities that described a broad range of physical activity behaviors (e.g., "weight lifter," "runner," "rollerblader") and modifications to their environments to support the changes in those behaviors (e.g., "minimal TV watcher," "taker of the long path," "goal setter"; see Chapter 3 for an in-depth analysis of the created doer identities for physical activity behaviors).

Predicting Physical Activity Behavior

To use doer identification in a way that would be meaningful for helping individuals engage in healthy lifestyle behaviors, is it important that self-as-doer identity can predict corresponding behavioral engagement in ways that existing factors do not. As such, Brouwer (n.d.) ran a hierarchical liner regression to determine whether self-as-doer identity could predict physical activity over and above existing motivational constructs (self-determinism, exercise motivations, exercise identity, and self-efficacy). Self-as-doer identity was a significant predictor, predicting an additional 1.9% of the variance in physical activity behaviors after controlling for the aforementioned constructs, $\Delta R^2 = .019$, $\Delta F (1, 197) = 5.77$, $p = .02$.[1] In this way, the self-as-doer can help us to understand why individuals may or may not engage in physical activity behaviors in ways that other constructs cannot.

Overall, findings suggest that doer identification has a unique role in health behavior engagement. Accordingly, researchers and interventionists can use the doer identity in ways that compliment and go beyond existing theories. If the self-as-doer identity can predict physical activity behaviors because, as the self-as-doer theory suggests, doer identification activates a cognitive process which provides motivation for engaging in a behavior, then it likely to be easily transferred to other important healthy lifestyle behaviors (e.g., weight loss, smoking cessation, safe sex practices). For example, if an existing intervention for weight loss is focused on increasing one's self-efficacy, yet the effects of the intervention are not as strong as desired, one might consider also addressing identity associated with doing weight loss behaviors. That is to say, seeing oneself as a "weight loser" or a "healthy weight maintainer" might provide the extra motivation needed to do the behavior and consequently see the desired results.

Relationships Among Doer Identification and Motivational Constructs

In addition to determining whether self-as-doer identity can predict physical activity behaviors beyond existing motivational constructs, the relationship between doer identity and exercise motivations, exercise identity, and self-efficacy for physical activity behaviors was also explored. Knowing how doer identification is related to these constructs can give researchers and interventionists a better picture of how to use it in promoting health behavior change.

Exercise Motivations

The relationship between the self-as-doer identity and motivations to exercise was examined in order to determine whether the self-as-doer identity was a unique motivational construct in predicting physical activity behaviors and how self-as-doer identity was related to various types of exercise motivations. The Exercise Motivations Index-2 (Markland & Ingledew, 1997) measures 14 different reasons for why people engage in physical activity. Doer identification was found to positively and significantly correlate with psychological motives (stress management, revitalization, enjoyment, and exercise as a challenge), social motives (social affiliation, social recognition, and competition needs), and fitness motives (strength, endurance, and nimbleness) for exercise. It was not correlated with body related motives (weight management and appearance) or health motives that emphasized negative outcomes (health pressures and ill-health avoidance). It was, however, positively correlated with the "positive health" health motive. Correlation coefficients can be found in Table 4.1.

Although most of the correlations were similar in strength (i.e., .18–.33), doer identity most strongly correlated with the challenge and affiliation motives. First, self-as-doer identity was specifically related to motivations

Table 4.1 Correlations between self-as-doer identity and exercise motivations

		Exercise motivations												
	Stress	*Revitalization*	*Enjoyment*	*Challenge*	*Social-recognition*	*Affiliation*	*Competition*	*Health pressures*	*Ill-health avoidance*	*Positive health*	*Weight management*	*Appearance*	*Strength and endurance*	*Nimbleness*
Self-as-doer	.21**	.21**	.26***	.33***	.22***	.30***	.23***	.06	.12	.17*	−.05	.06	.27***	.18**

* p <.05;
**p <.01;
*** p < .001.

that focus on physical activity as a means of having a personal challenge to face or developing personal skills and exploring limits of one's body. These motivations are clearly in line with the self-as-doer theory in that doer identity is focused on behavior based upon goals that promote personal betterment. Second, the self-as-doer was related to affiliation motives, which corresponds to wanting to include others in physical activities. For instance, individuals exercise to spend time with friends, to have fun being active with other people, and to make new friends. Although it is argued that the self-as-doer is primarily focused on the self, it may be that doer identification is strengthened by sharing that identity with others or that by participating in physical activity with others, one begins to take cues from the social environment and modify their self-concept as the doer of their behaviors accordingly. Overall, if one were to develop an intervention for physical activity, it would be valuable to consider how doer identity might promote these forms of motivations or that individuals with such motivations might be more likely to develop doer identities related to physical activity.

As it relates to motivations for physical activity behaviors, the self-as-doer is theoretically supported in that it is associated with diverse motives (i.e., psychology, social, and fitness) that involve more self-determined behaviors (e.g., enjoyment, challenge, skill improvement, affiliation, positive health etc.). That the self-as-doer was not associated with motivations that emphasize negative outcomes like ill-health avoidance or external motivations like health pressures further supports the notion that doer identity is focused on internal motivation for actively engaging in physical behavior. Additionally, the lack of relationships with appearance and weight maintenance might suggest that doer identity is associated with linking the self with the behavior and not just the self-concept. Both appearance and weight maintenance motivations are primarily reflective of the image of the self (e.g., "look more attractive," "have a good body," to stay slim") rather than a performing a behavior. In sum, the self-as-doer identity is related to diverse exercise motivations that align with more self-determined behaviors, but is arguably a distinct form of motivation for physical activity behaviors.

Exercise Identity

Exercise-specific identity has been associated with greater frequency of physical activity behaviors (Grant, Hogg, & Crano, 2015; Miller, Ogletree, & Welshimer, 2002; Reifsteck, Gill, & Labban, 2016; Strachan, Brawley, Spink, & Jung, 2009; Wilson & Muon, 2008). Exercise identity, as conceptualized by Anderson and Cychosz (1994) in their Exercise Identity Scale and later modified by Wilson and Muon (2008), is comprised of identity roles (e.g., "Others see me as someone who exercises regularly") and exercise beliefs (e.g., "I have numerous goals related to exercising"). Although theoretically similar, the self-as-doer is different in that it represents the active agent of the behavior, not just the roles one might have or the beliefs one might hold about exercise behaviors. What makes the self-as-doer unique is the connecting of one's self-concept with the physical activity behavior. To assess the degree of overlap between exercise identity and a self-as-doer identity, the self-as-doer was correlated with exercise identity (Brouwer, n.d.). Results demonstrated that the self-as-doer identity was positively and significantly correlated with the role identity (.39, *p* < .001) and exercise beliefs (r = .29, *p* < .001) subscales of the Exercise Identity Scale. That doer identification was positively correlated with both subscales suggests that doer identification is associated with both exercise roles and beliefs. That is, a stronger doer identity is related to a stronger likelihood of endorsing exercise roles and participatory beliefs about exercise. However, that the correlation was only a medium effect supports the idea that the self-as-doer is not the same construct as exercise roles and beliefs.

Self-Efficacy

Self-efficacy, the belief in one's ability to perform a behavior, plays a vital role in predicting health behaviors (Bandura, 1998; Luszczynska et al., 2016; Nezami et al., 2016; Sheeran et al., 2016), especially physical activity behaviors (Olander et al., 2013; Higgins, Middleton, Winner, & Janelle, 2014; Shieh, Weaver, Hanna, Newsome, & Mogos, 2015). To ascertain the relationship between self-as-doer identity and self-efficacy for general physical activity and self-efficacy for overcoming barriers related to physical activity, correlations were computed. Results demonstrated that stronger doer identification was associated with greater self-efficacy for engaging in physical activity behaviors (r = .17, *p* = .01) and for overcoming barriers to physical activity behaviors (r = .25, *p* < .001). In general, results demonstrate that doer identity is positively associated with the degree of confidence one feels about their abilities to engage in physical activity and to overcome barriers associated with physical activity. Again, results affirm the self-as-doer theory in that the self-as-doer identity is positively related to other factors which have a predictive relationship with physical activity behaviors.

In sum, the self-as-doer identity can predict physical activity above and beyond other motivational constructs and is associated with exercise identity roles and beliefs, and self-efficacy for both physical activity behaviors in general and for overcoming barriers. The generally positive and moderate relationships that self-as-doer identity has with exercise identity, self-efficacy, and motivations for exercise suggests that self-as-doer identity is a distinct factor that can be used alongside of these constructs without being superfluous and therefore strengthening the ability to determine what contributes to health behavior change and maintenance. Although our conclusions about these relationships are specific to physical activity behaviors, the nature and theory of the self-as-doer identity suggests that such findings can be generalized to other healthy lifestyle behaviors (e.g., weight loss, safe sex practices, smoking cessation, etc.)

It is important to note, however, that this work is limited in that it is correlational and it is not possible to determine whether engaging in physical activity increases one's identification with a behavior or whether the development of an identity as the doer of one's behavior causes behavior change. In an effort to determine whether manipulating the self-as-doer identity could lead to corresponding behavior change, Brouwer and Mosack (2015) developed an intervention aimed at activating self-as-doer identities and tested whether it would cause a change in diet behaviors and whether this behavior change could be maintained.

Self-as-Doer Identity and Diet Behaviors (The Healthy Eating Study)

The self-as-doer intervention was developed from the idea that conceptualizing the degree to which one identifies with goals and behavior related to certain behavior change (e.g., more fruit consumption) and discussing the discrepancies between one's current identification (i.e., a poor fruit eater) and what it might take to define oneself to a stronger degree in relation to the behavior in question (e.g., purchase more fruits to become a better fruit eater) could be a means to bring about change in behavioral intention and behavior (O'Keefe, 2002). The processes whereby individuals identify goals related to healthy eating and transform those goals into identity statements (i.e., the self-as-doer) was projected to have the potential to activate existing self-representations related to healthy eating. Furthermore, the cognitive process of conceptualizing what it means to be a "healthy eater" can bring about greater identification with different, more health consistent behaviors which may consequently promote behavior change. Therefore, the primary objectives of the self-as-doer intervention were to assist participants with developing goals related to healthy eating behaviors, transforming those goals into self-as-doer identity statements, and then reflecting on the degree to which doer identities were descriptive of oneself.

For the experimental evaluation of the intervention, participants were asked to complete the self-as-doer measure and then answer a few questions related to the doer identities they created (Brouwer & Mosack, 2015). As was described in the physical activity study, prior to competing the self-as-doer measure, participants reviewed educational information. For this study, however, it was nutritional education in the form of pamphlets and brochures created by the United States Department of Agriculture (USDA, 2010a, 2010b, 2010c). As before, the educational material served as both a prime and a resource to assist participants in generating appropriate goals; however, for this study, the goals were specific to healthy eating behaviors. Although the focus of the study was to measure the degree of change in fruit, vegetable, whole grain, low-fat dairy, and sugar-sweetened beverage consumption, participants were not restricted in the types of healthy eating goals that they could create (see Chapter 3 for details on created doer phrases). The methods for creating doer identities and rating those doer identities in terms of how well each created identity described the participant were similar to that described previously in the physical activity study.

Upon completion of the self-as-doer measure, the interviewer then began the process of helping the participant reflect on the degree to which doer identities were consistent with their current self-concept and, if not, how one would go about enhancing that consistency. For this process (and as has been described previously in Brouwer & Mosack, 2015), the interviewer selected one of the created doer identities and asked participants to envision themselves as the doer of the "-er" phrase they constructed. For example, the researcher might say, "Picture yourself being a fruit eater. What would that look like?" Participants were then allowed time to verbally describe the form that this doer identity took for them. After this description, the researcher then identified how the participant rated that particular identity and asked them how they could see themselves as that doer identity to a greater degree in subsequent weeks. For example, the interviewer would say, "I see that you rated yourself as a 'fruit eater' as a 2 (does not describe me well). What would it take in this next week and beyond this next week to see yourself as a fruit eater to a greater degree, say a 4 or a 5 instead of a 2?" This process was repeated for 3 or 4 of the created doer identities. Participants were then provided with a verbal summary of the task and encouraged to think about their doer identities as they made diet choices in later weeks (Brouwer & Mosack, 2015).

The outcomes of the study were measured by having participants complete food diaries 1 week before the intervention, 1 week after the intervention and then again 1 month following the intervention. The study lasted approximately 6 weeks and a healthy diet was operationalized as increases in one's consumption of fruits, vegetables, whole grains, and low-fat dairy and a reduction in sugar-sweetened beverage consumption. The diets of those who received the self-as-doer intervention were compared to a nutrition education group (i.e., those who read the aforementioned USDA nutrition education pamphlets) and a control group (i.e., those who received no intervention; see Brouwer & Mosack, 2015 for a detailed description of the study hypotheses and procedures).

Dietary Change Results

Results demonstrated that the self-as-doer intervention was an effective tool to promote maintenance of overall healthy eating behaviors. Participants who completed the intervention had significantly[2] higher rates of overall healthy food consumption at the one-month follow-up than did those who received only nutrition education ((t[116]= 2.19, p = .09) and those in the control group (t[116] = 2.53, p = .04). The effect of the intervention for specific food groups was mixed. There were no specific effects for fruit and vegetable consumption, but there were some significant changes across time and significant differences between groups for whole grain, low-fat dairy, and sugar-sweetened beverage consumption (see Figure 4.1).

Participants who completed the self-as-doer intervention significantly increased their whole grain consumption from baseline to post-intervention.

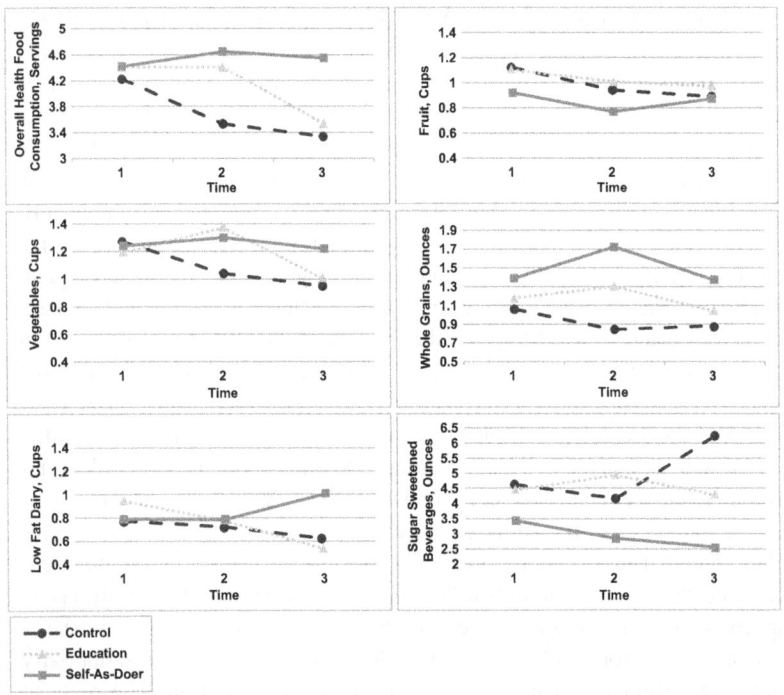

Figure 4.1 Change across time and differences among groups for overall and food-group specific health food consumption

Source: From "Motivating health diet behaviors: The self-as-doer identity" by A. M. Brouwer and K. E. Mosack, 2015, *Self and Identity, 14*, p. 648.Copyright [2015] by Taylor & Francis. Reprinted with permission.

This increase, coinciding with a significant decrease in whole grain consumption in the control group, led to a significant difference between those who had the self-as-doer intervention and those in the control group one week after the intervention, $t(116)= 3.40$, $p = 003$. There was, however, a significant decrease in whole grain consumption for the self-as-doer intervention group, returning their consumption back to baseline rates at the one-month follow-up time period. For low-fat dairy consumption, participants who received the intervention had significant increases in their consumption rates between the week after the intervention and the one-month follow-up, $t[116] = 2.26$, $p = .08$. At one-month follow-up, those who received the self-as-doer intervention had significantly higher low-fat dairy consumption than those who received nutrition education ($t[116] = 2.62$, $p = .03$) and lower sugar-sweetened beverage consumption than did those in the control group, $t(116) = 2.63$, $p = .03$.

Overall, the findings demonstrated that although the self-as-doer intervention did not increase healthy food consumption, it did cause participants to maintain a higher level of healthy eating behaviors compared to those who only received nutrition education and those who received no intervention (Brouwer & Mosack, 2015). As such, using the self-as-doer intervention could play and important role in promoting the maintenance of other healthy lifestyle behaviors. For example, perhaps an individual is considering losing weight or maintaining weight loss but has struggled to do so. It may be that adopting an identity as a "weight loser" or a "healthy weight maintainer" and then reflecting on how one could see oneself as that identity to a stronger degree could create the added motivation needed to not just change but also maintain these health behaviors. The same could be said for smoking behaviors. If an individual wants to quit smoking, but is facing barriers in being able to maintain a reduction in smoking, developing goals and corresponding self-as-doer identities to reduce and eventually quit smoking (e.g., "smoking reducer," "one cigarette a day smoker," "smoking quitter") could provide the added motivation to overcome the barriers that initially prevented the behavior change and that caused relapse in the unwanted behavior.

The self-as-doer intervention caused participants to maintain their overall healthy eating behaviors but had less consistent effects for specific food groups. Participants may have focused on changing one or two diet behaviors at a time, making finding statistical significance for all diet behaviors difficult (Brouwer & Mosack, 2015). As a result, further interventions might focus more specifically on addressing certain foods rather than on the broader behavior of eating a healthy diet. The specificity might help individuals focus on a single identity that can be translated more successfully into behavior change. Participants may have also had insufficient knowledge about nutrition to increase their healthy food consumption in a statistically measurable degree. One participant, for example, chose to make dietary changes related to fruit and whole grain consumption by drinking more fruit juice and eating certain granola bars because the packaging advertised that they were made from whole grains. Unfortunately the juice she chose contained only 10% fruit juice and the amount of whole grains in each granola bar was very small, only 0.25 ounces. As such, her behavior changed, but not in a sufficiently measurable form (Brouwer & Mosack, 2015). One could argue that for cases such as these, the self-as-doer intervention did have a meaningful change in health behavior. Going forward with the intervention, it may be important to provide adequate and accurate nutritional information so that participants are clear on what constitutes a measurable change in each of their behavioral goals and what pitfalls are common when making healthy food decisions (e.g., false advertising). For example, one could provide a list of foods which have the highest whole grain amounts or vegetables that are considered to be more highly nutritious than others (e.g., dark green and orange vegetables vs. lettuce).

Results of the Intervention Impact

Participants' responses, both solicited and unsolicited, to the self-as-doer intervention were also recorded in an effort to better understand the most salient parts of the self-as-doer intervention (Brouwer & Mosack, 2015). First, participants reported adopting their doer identities and using them to make healthy diet choices. In an unsolicited email one participant described how she was "excited to become a 'leafy vegetable eater'," a doer-identity phrase she created at the time of the self-as-doer intervention. Another participant, without prompting, wrote the created doer identities next to foods that supported that identity in her food diaries. For example, she wrote "veggie grabber" next to foods such as celery and carrots that she ate. Another participant who saw herself as a "quinoa eater" also found that part of that identity includes sharing her recipe discoveries with others. After the lab visit where she created doer identities, she brought in a sample of quinoa and tips on how best to serve it as part of one's meal.

Participants also reported how thinking about doer identities helped them to make healthier diet choices. For example, one participant described how she was at a vending machine preparing to get her usual sugar-sweetened beverage, but before making the selection, she thought to herself, "no, I'm a 'less sugar drinker' (a doer identity she had created in the intervention) and should chose a diet beverage instead." The identity as a "less sugar drinker" led her to then choose a diet drink rather than her habitual choice of a sugar-sweetened drink. Defining oneself according to a doer identity also led participants to make healthy choices, even when it was not the preferred choice. For example, at a follow-up visit, one participant inquired about the amount of vegetables in a vegetarian burger. Upon finding out that there was only about one-quarter cup servings of vegetables in the burger she said, "You mean I choked down that veggie burger instead of a hot dog for only a quarter cup of veggies?" (Brouwer & Mosack, 2015).

Overall, the self-as-doer intervention was effective in getting individuals to think about themselves as the doer of their behaviors and from both qualitative and quantitative results, the intervention demonstrates how a motivational identity can promote the maintenance of healthy eating behaviors. Although not all food-group specific healthy eating behaviors were changed over the course of the study, the findings support previous research (Brouwer & Mosack, 2012; Houser-Marko & Sheldon, 2006; RiseSheeran, & Hukkelberg, 2010; Stryker & Burke, 2000) and demonstrate how the self-as-doer identity can be activated through a simple environmental intervention to consequently influence health behavior change and maintenance related to healthy eating.

Conclusion

In this chapter the utility of the self-as-doer in healthy, non-clinical populations has been discussed. Health behavior change and maintenance are difficult, but the self-as-doer provides a motivational identity that can be used to overcome barriers to promote sustaining health behavior enactment. The use of the self-as-doer identity within the context of physical activity behaviors and diet demonstrates that, indeed, a doer identification can predict health behaviors and even promote the maintenance of that behavior. That the self-as-doer is about processing how one sees oneself as the doer of his or her goals gives it universal applicability. The steps of creating goals, transforming those goals into doer statements, and then reflecting on the degree to which on could see oneself as that doer to a stronger degree can be applied to most any healthy lifestyle behavior. The research reviewed in this chapter supports the self-as-doer theory that linking a self-concept to a behavior in order to conceptualize oneself as the doer of one's behavior can have an effect on health behavior, especially maintenance of that behavior. Therefore, there is promise in using the self-as-doer in diverse health behaviors among non-clinical populations. Given its widespread applicability, the self-as-doer could be used, for example, to promote safer sex practices, better sleep habits, participating in disease-prevention screenings, and managing stress in healthy populations. This approach can also be useful to promote improve health behaviors and manage chronic conditions within clinical populations too. To that end, I now turn to discussing how the self-as-doer identity can be used as a disease management tool.

Notes

1. Additional statistical details are available from the author.
2. Bonferroni corrections were performed for all follow-up analyses to control for type I errors. Given that the original study was designed as a pilot study, significance criteria were set at $p = .10$.

References

Agboola, S., Mcneill, A., Coleman, T., & Leonardi, B. J. (2010). A systematic review of the effectiveness of smoking relapse prevention interventions for abstinent smokers. *Addiction, 105,* 1362–1380. doi: 10.1111/j.1360-0443.2010.02996.x

Anderson, D. F., & Cychosz, C. M. (1994). Development of an exercise identity scale. *Perceptual and Motor Skills, 78*(3, Pt 1), 747–751. doi: 10.2466/pms.1994.78.3.747

Avenell, A., Broom, J., Brown, T. J., Poobalan, A., Aucott, L., Stearns, S. C., . . . Grant, A. M. (2004). Systematic review of the long-term effects and economic consequences of treatments for obesity and implications for health improvement. *Health Technology Assessment, 8*(21), 1–182.

Bandura, A. (1998). Health promotion from the perspective of social cognitive theory. *Psychology and Health, 13,* 623–649. doi: 10.1080/08870449808407422

Barnidge, E. K., Radvanyi, C., Duggan, K., Motton, F., Wiggs, I., Baker, E. A., & Brownson, R. C. (2013). Understanding and addressing barriers to implementation of environmental and policy interventions to support physical activity and healthy eating in rural communities. *Journal of Rural Health, 29*(1), 97–105. doi: 10.1111/j.1748-0361.2012.00431.x

Brouwer, A. M. (n.d.). *Predicting physical activity with identity: The self-as-doer identity.* Unpublished manuscript.

Brouwer, A. M., & Mosack, K. E. (2015). Motivating health diet behaviors: The self-as-doer identity. *Self and Identity, 14,* 638–653. doi: 10.1080/15298868.2015.1043335

Center for Disease Control (2015). *The benefits of physical activity.* Retrieved from www.cdc.gov/physicalactivity/basics/pa-health/

Department of Health and Human Services (2008). *2008 physical activity guidelines for Americans.* Retrieved from https://health.gov/paguidelines/pdf/paguide.pdf

Dombrowski, S. U., Knittle, K., Avenell, A., Araujo-Soares, V., & Sniehotta, F. F. (2014). Long-term maintenance of weight loss in obese adults: A systematic review of randomised controlled trials of nonsurgical weight loss maintenance interventions with meta-analyses. *British Medical Journal, 348,* g2646. doi: 10.1136/bmj.g2646

Fjeldsoe, B., Neuhaus, M., Winkler, E., & Eakin, E. (2011). Systematic review of maintenance of behavior change following physical activity and dietary interventions. *Health Psychology, 30*(1), 99–109. doi: 10.1037/a0021974

Ford, E. S., Zhao, G., Tsai, J., & Li, C. (2011). Low-risk lifestyle behaviors and all-cause mortality: Findings from the National Health and Nutrition Examination Survey III Mortality Study. *American Journal of Public Health, 101*(10), 1922–1929. doi: 10.2105/AJPH.2011.300167

Foster, G. D., Wyatt, H. R., Hill, J. O., Makris, A. P., Rosenbaum, D. L., Brill, C., . . . Klein, S. (2010). Weight and metabolic outcomes after 2 years on a low-carbohydrate versus low-fat diet: A randomized trial. *Annals of Internal Medicine, 153*, 147–157. doi: 10.7326/0003-4819-153-3-201008030-00005

Grant, F., Hogg, M. A., & Crano, W. D. (2015). Yes, we can: Physical activity and group identification among healthy adults. *Journal of Applied Social Psychology, 45*(7), 383–390. doi: 10.1111/jasp.12305

Higgins, T. J., Middleton, K. R., Winner, L., & Janelle, C. M. (2014). Physical activity interventions differentially affect exercise task and barrier self-efficacy: A meta-analysis. *Health Psychology, 33*(8), 891–903. doi: 10.1037/a0033864

Houser-Marko, L., & Sheldon, K. M. (2006). Motivating behavioral persistence: The self-as-doer construct. *Personality and Social Psychology Bulletin, 32*, 1037–1049. doi: 10.1177/0146167206287974

Jones, M., Lewis, S., Parrott, S., Wormall, S., & Coleman, T. (2016). Re-starting smoking in the postpartum period after receiving a smoking cessation intervention: A systematic review. *Addiction, 111*(6), 981–990. doi: 10.1111/add.13309

Joseph, R. P., Ainsworth, B. E., Keller, C., & Dodgson, J. E. (2015). Barriers to physical activity among African American women: An integrative review of the literature. *Women & Health, 55*(6), 679–699. doi: 10.1080/03630242.2015.1039184

Kroeze, W., Werkman, A., & Brug, J. (2006). A systematic review of randomized trials on the effectiveness of computer-tailored education on physical activity and dietary behaviors. *Annals of Behavioral Medicine, 31*, 205–223. doi: 10.1207/s15324796abm3103_2

Loef, M., & Walach, H. (2012). The combined effects of healthy lifestyle behaviors on all cause mortality: A systematic review and meta-analysis. *Preventive Medicine: An International Journal Devoted to Practice and Theory, 55*(3), 163–170. doi: 10.1016/j.ypmed.2012.06.017

Luszczynska, A., Horodyska, K., Zarychta, K., Liszewska, N., Knoll, N., & Scholz, U. (2016). Planning and self-efficacy interventions encouraging replacing energy-dense foods intake with fruit and vegetable: A longitudinal experimental study. *Psychology & Health, 31*(1), 40–64. doi: 10.1080/08870446.2015.1070156

Macniven, R., Pye, V., Merom, D., Milat, A., Monger, C., Bauman, A., & van der Ploeg, H. (2014). Barriers and enablers to physical activity among older Australians who want to increase their physical activity levels. *Journal of Physical Activity & Health, 11*(7), 1420–1429. doi: 10.1123/jpah.2012–0096

Markland, D., & Ingledew, D. K. (1997). The measurement of exercise motives: Factorial validity and invariance across gender of a revised exercise motivations inventory. *British Journal of Health Psychology, 2*, 361–376. doi: 10.1111/j.2044-8287.1997.tb00549.x

Martins, J., Marques, A., Sarmento, H., & da Costa, F. C. (2015). Adolescents' perspectives on the barriers and facilitators of physical activity: A systematic review of qualitative studies. *Health Education Research, 30*(5), 742–755. doi: 10.1093/her/cyv042

Miller, K. M., Ogletree, R. J., & Welshimer, K. (2002). Impact of activity behaviors in physical activity identity and self-efficacy. *American Journal of Health Behavior*, *26*, 323–330. doi: 10.5993/AJHB.26.5.1

Nezami, B. T., Lang, W., Jakicic, J. M., Davis, K. K., Polzien, K., Rickman, A. D., . . . Tate, D. F. (2016). The effect of self-efficacy on behavior and weight in a behavioral weight-loss intervention. *Health Psychology*, *35*(7), 714–722. doi: 10.1037/hea0000378

Nicklett, E. J., Semba, R. D., Xue, Q., Tian, J., Sun, K., Cappola, A. R., . . . Fried, L. P. (2012). Fruit and vegetable intake, physical activity, and mortality in older community-dwelling women. *Journal of the American Geriatrics Society*, *60*(5), 862–868. doi: 10.1111/j.1532-5415.2012.03924.x

O'Keefe, D. J. (2002). *Persuasion: Theory and research*. Beverly Hills, CA: Sage.

Olander, E. K., Fletcher, H., Williams, S., Lou, A., Turner, A., & French, D. P. (2013). What are the most effective techniques in changing obese individuals' physical activity self-efficacy and behaviour: A systematic review and meta-analysis. *International Journal of Behavioral Nutrition and Physical Activity*, *10*. doi: 10.1186/1479-5868-10-29

Reifsteck, E. J., Gill, D. L., & Labban, J. D. (2016). "Athletes" and "exercisers": Understanding identity, motivation, and physical activity participation in former college athletes. *Sport, Exercise, and Performance Psychology*, *5*(1), 25–38. doi: 10.1037/spy0000046

Riekert, K. A., Ockene, J. K., & Pbert, L. (Eds.). (2014). *The handbook of health behavior change*. New York: Springer Publishing.

Rise, J., Sheeran, P., & Hukkelberg, S. (2010). The role of self-identity in the theory of planned behavior: A meta-analysis. *Journal of Applied Social Psychology*, *40*, 1085–1105. doi: 10.1111/j.1559-1816.2010.00611.x/pdf

Sheeran, P., Maki, A., Montanaro, E., Avishai-Yitshak, A., Bryan, A., Klein, W. P., . . . Rothman, A. J. (2016). The impact of changing attitudes, norms, and self-efficacy on health-related intentions and behavior: A meta-analysis. *Health Psychology*, *35*(11), 1178–1188. doi: 10.1037/hea0000387

Shieh, C., Weaver, M. T., Hanna, K. M., Newsome, K., & Mogos, M. (2015). Association of self-efficacy and self-regulation with nutrition and exercise behaviors in a community sample of adults. *Journal of Community Health Nursing*, *32*(4), 199–211. doi: 10.1080/07370016.2015.1087262

Spruijt-Metz, D., Hekler, E., Saranummi, N., Intille, S., Korhonen, I., Nilsen, W., . . . Pavel, M. (2015). Building new computational models to support health behavior change and maintenance: New opportunities in behavioral research. *Translational Behavioral Medicine*, *5*(3), 335–346. doi: 10.1007/s13142-015-0324-1

Strachan, S. M., Brawley, L. R., Spink, K. S., & Jung, M. E. (2009). Strength of exercise identity and identity-exercise consistency. *Journal of Health Psychology*, *14*, 1196–1206. doi: 10.1177/1359105309346340

Stryker, S., & Burke, P. J. (2000). The past, present, and future of identity theory. *Social Psychology Quarterly*, *63*, 284–297. Retrieved from www.jstor.org/stable/2695840

Thorpe, R. J., Wilson-Frederick, S. M., Bowie, J. V., Coa, K., Clay, O. J., LaVeist, T. A., & Whitfield, K. E. (2013). Health behaviors and all-cause mortality in African

American men. *American Journal of Men's Health, 7*(4, Suppl.), 8S–18S. doi: 10.1177/1557988313487552

U.S. Department of Agriculture (2010a). *Let's eat for the health of it.* Retrieved from www.choosemyplate.gov/sites/default/files/audiences/DG2010Brochure.pdf

U.S. Department of Agriculture (2010b). *Build a healthy meal.* Retrieved from www.choosemyplate.gov/sites/default/files/tentips/DGTipsheet38BuildHealthy MealtimeHabits_0.pdf

U.S. Department of Agriculture (2010c). *Choose MyPlate 10 tips to a great plate.* Retrieved from www.choosemyplate.gov/sites/default/files/tentips/DGTipsheet1 ChooseMyPlate.pdf

Wilson, P. M., & Muon, S. (2008). Psychometric properties of the exercise identity scale in a university sample. *International Journal of Sport and Exercise Psychology, 6*(2), 115–131. doi: 10.1080/1612197X.2008.96718

5 Self-as-Doer Identity and Health Behavior Change Within Clinical Populations

Amanda M. Brouwer and Katie E. Mosack

The self-as-doer identity can be used to promote health behavior change in clinical populations, particularly given the unique set of challenges that individuals within these populations face. In the following chapter, the attributes of the self-as-doer identity that make it relevant to clinical populations will be discussed and specific examples and research within the context of individuals with diabetes will be used to support the role of the self-as-doer in health promotion for other clinical populations.

Individuals with chronic illness represent a unique population when promoting health behavior change because disease management often requires a set of prescribed behaviors that can be arduous and burdensome. Moreover motivation for maintaining behavior is often difficult, as evidenced by low adherence and high dropout rates in traditional behavior change programs (Crutzen, Viechtbauer, Spigt, & Kotz, 2015; de Bruin, McCambridge, & Prins, 2015; Dumville, Torgerson, & Hewitt, 2006). Clinical populations, compared to non-clinical populations, are also more likely to see the need for behavior change as a way to avoid negative consequences of an illness (e.g., heart failure, high cholesterol, vision problems, etc.), rather than acquiring something from engaging in a new health behavior (e.g., lose weight to look better, run to increase cardiovascular strength). For clinical populations, this loss-framed, avoidance orientation (compared with the gain-framed, approach orientation) creates a different perspective to disease management and health behavior enactment which may consequently affect motivation. Elliot (2006) describes avoidance motivation as simply trying to survive and, as such, can lead to behaviors which are less likely to be enacted and maintained overtime. Approach motivation, on the other hand, can be described as trying to thrive and is associated with greater adherence to health behavior enactment and maintenance (Taylor, 2013; Williams, Haskard-Zolnierek, & Dimatteo, 2014) and might be more relevant for behavior change among relatively healthy people.

Given the added difficulty of behavior change for clinical populations as a result the aforementioned effects of behavior change in the context of an illness, the self-as-doer identity might be particularly well-suited to provide the needed motivation for behavior change in a way that can help individuals thrive. The self-as-doer identity can serve as a source of motivation especially when the behavior is difficult and the benefits of engaging in that behavior are not reinforcing. Consider, for example, an individual who takes medication for high blood pressure. Medication adherence might fluctuate relative to the experience of unpleasant side effects like rashes, feeling weak, sleepiness, etc. Breaking out in a visible rash could be more aversive to an individual than having high blood pressure and therefore medication might not be taken as prescribed. Endorsing one's identity as a "medication taker," for example, might provide the motivation to go beyond the side effects and increase adherence to the medication regimen. Furthermore, the self-as-doer identity is defined by doing a behavior and not being rewarded by the consequences of the behavior. As such, the identity as the doer of a behavior provides a form of motivation that might be uniquely suited to promote and maintain health behaviors that are challenging. Likewise, the self-as-doer identity is particularly applicable for disease management that is chronic and requires a degree of personal responsibility to enact behaviors (e.g., taking medication, getting regular exercise, following a specific diet, etc.) because it is a self-concept rooted in personal goal setting. Finally, having a self-as-doer identity encourages an approach-framed motivation because it requires that individuals think of themselves as the doer of the behavior—the enactor and the active agent that is fulfilling a goal rather than avoiding a negative consequence. As such, clinical populations may be better served if motivation for behavior change can be developed through seeing themselves as the doers of their behaviors.

To better understand how the self-as-doer can operate within clinical populations, consider individuals with diabetes. Diabetes is a chronic, taxing disease requiring strict adherence to medical regimens and regular practices of self-care behaviors in order to maintain adequate glycemic control and consequently good health (American Diabetes Association [ADA], 2016). General guidelines for maintaining good health include healthy eating, being active, monitoring blood glucose levels, taking medication, problem solving, risk reduction, and healthy coping (ADA, 2016; Shirvastava, Shrivastava, & Ramasamy, 2013). Each of these behaviors requires that the individual take responsibility for enacting the behavior. The health care professional is not able to monitor blood glucose or make healthy diet choices for the individual on a daily basis. As such, self-care management for a chronic illness like diabetes requires personal responsibility and identification with the disease and the behaviors required to manage the disease.

Given that the self-as-doer identity is an identity focused on the self (versus others) and engenders an identity as the doer of behaviors regardless of reinforcement, thinking of oneself as the doer of self-care management behaviors—a "blood sugar checker" or a "medication taker"—can provide the motivation needed to enact and sustain these required behaviors. To empirically determine the role of doer identification in diabetes self-care care management, Brouwer (2008) and Brouwer and Mosack (2012, 2013) conducted a series of studies to explore how self-as-doer identity can be measured relative to diabetes self-care behaviors and whether it can predict diabetes self-care behaviors and overall diabetes health. A discussion of these studies and the outcomes of each will serve as a foundation for understanding how the self-as-doer works in a clinical population and the degree to which it can be generalized to other similar clinical populations.

Diabetes Health Pilot Study

Brouwer (2008) first conducted a pilot study to determine whether self-as-doer identity was correlated with diabetes self-care behaviors and whether it could predict diabetes self-care behaviors above and beyond existing constructs that have been found predict diabetes self-care behaviors. The researcher recruited 97 people with type 1 and type 2 diabetes to complete a set of questionnaires assessing diabetes-specific self-efficacy, social support, outcome expectancies, self-care agency, and the frequencies to which diabetes self-care behaviors were performed. Participants also completed the self-as-doer measure with instructions to identity goals specific to their diabetes self-care management. Without assistance from an interviewer, participants created goals and corresponding doer identities that reflected general recommendations for diabetes self-care management (e.g., eating healthy, getting regular exercise, blood glucose monitoring, taking medication, etc.; for a more detailed analysis of goals and created doer identities see Chapter 3). In regards to the predictive relationship between self-as-doer identity and diabetes self-care behaviors, the researcher found that diabetes-specific self-efficacy and self-as-doer identity were significant predictors of diabetes self-care behaviors. Self-as-doer identity accounted uniquely for 3.8% of the variance in diabetes self-care behaviors, ($\Delta R^2 = .038$, $\Delta F(70) = 5.61$, $p = .021$) whereas outcome expectancies, social support, and self-care agency were not predictive of diabetes self-care behaviors.

Because the self-as-doer identity predicted self-care behaviors, researchers were able to demonstrate that developing an identity as the doer of a behavior that is consistent with one's health care goals is beneficial for motivating self-care behaviors. However, the way in which self-as-doer identity is measured, particularly in the pilot study with individuals who have diabetes, may be somewhat limited when assessing those with chronic illnesses. In the diabetes health pilot study, instructions for the self-as-doer measure were to create goals and, subsequently, doer identities related to diabetes self-care management. In this form, participants could create idiosyncratic doer identities that may not directly reflect their chronic illness-specific self-care management. As such, a doer identity for diabetes-specific self-care behaviors could vary from individual to individual. In cases where self-care management recommendations are generally consistent across individuals, as in the case of diabetes, researchers, interventionists, and health care professionals might benefit from using a standardized measure with doer identities specific to the self-care management behaviors recommended for those with the disease. This form of measuring doer identity would provide a standardized way to measure, modify, and develop interventions focused on doer identities that are appropriate for the self-care management of the specific chronic illness. Consequently, for the next study researchers did just this; they developed and tested a diabetes-specific measure of doer identification.

Development of the Self-as-Doer-Diabetes Measure

The Self-as-Doer-Diabetes scale (SD-D; Brouwer & Mosack, 2013) is a 42-item scale that measures the degree to which individuals with diabetes see themselves as the doer of diabetes self-care behaviors. The SD-D was created from 522 doer identities that persons with both type 1 and type 2 diabetes created in the aforementioned diabetes health pilot study (Brouwer, 2008; for an analysis of those doer identities see Chapter 3). Using themes generated from these doer identities (e.g., diet, exercise, glucose monitoring, medication taking, sleep, and stress) explicit but inclusive self-as-doer identity statements for diabetes self-care behaviors were created for the measure. To ensure accuracy of the doer identity theory and adequate representation of diabetes self-care behaviors, the created items were shared with experts (i.e., 2 others who have diabetes, 4 diabetes nurse educators, and the authors of the self-as-doer theory) and their feedback was incorporated to further refine the measure. As in the original self-as-doer measure, for the SD-D participants are prompted to respond to each item on a scale of 1 (*does not describe me well at all*) to 5 (*describes me very well*) on the degree to which they see themselves as each doer identity (See Appendix 5.1 for the SD-D measure).

To assess the degree to which the SD-D measured self-as-doer identity and not other related psychological constructs, the SD-D was correlated with diabetes-specific constructs such as illness perception, self-determinism, self-efficacy, locus of control, and outcome expectancies. Furthermore, if the SD-D is measuring self-as-doer identity, then it should also predict diabetes self-care behaviors, as it has in past research. Consequently, analyses were run to determine whether the SD-D could predict diabetes self-care behaviors and adequate hemoglobin A1c (HbA1c; HbA1c is a measure of average glucose in the blood). Good diabetes control is established by having an HbA1c less than 7.1% (ADA, 2016), above and beyond demographics and related psychological variables.

To test the measure, 355 individuals with diabetes (207 with type 1 and 148 with type 2) completed a survey with questions about demographics, the aforementioned psychological variables, and the SD-D. In an analysis of the factor structure, seven subscales were meaningful interpreted as the following doer identities: (1) Blood Glucose Monitor, (2) Physical Activity Doer, (3) Active Health Care Participator, (4) Medication/Insulin Regulator, (5) Secondary Care Doer, (6) Stress Regulator, and (7) Food/Diet Follower. Doer identities, for the most part, reflected recommendations provided by the ADA—to monitor blood sugars, get regular physical activity, take medication, and eat a healthy diet. However, the doer identities participants constructed reflected behaviors that might seem secondary to diabetes self-management objectives (e.g., being an active participator in health care decision making, keeping health care appointments). Yet an improvement in these behaviors and the degree to which one might identify with them can lead to better overall medical adherence thereby enhancing the value of seeing oneself as the doer of not just the primary self-management behaviors, but also ones that are considered secondary or supplemental.

The measure and subscales were reliable (Cronbach's alpha for the overall SD-D was .93 and subscales ranged from .72-.89), all SD-D subscales moderately to strongly correlated with one another, and the SD-D was positively and moderately to strongly correlated with autonomous and controlled motivation, internal autonomy, outcome expectancies, self-efficacy, and diabetes self-care behaviors. (See Brouwer & Mosack, 2013 for detailed statistical analyses.) Consequently the measure was deemed valid and reliable.

To assess whether the SD-D was actually a representation of self-as-doer identity, it was used to predict diabetes self-care behaviors and HbA1c. Using the SD-D, self-as-doer identity specific to diabetes self-care behavior was a significant predictor of diet ($R^2 = .04$, $F(1,120) = 9.25$, $p < .01$), physical activity ($R^2 = .08$, $F(1,124) = 15.15$, $p < .001$), medication ($R^2 = .03$, $F(1,126) = 4.79$, $p < .01$), and foot care behaviors ($R^2 = .04$, $F(1,126) = 7.33$, $p < .01$) for persons with type 1 diabetes above and beyond demographics and psychological variables. Self-as-doer identity was also a significant predictor of diet ($R^2 = .10$, $F(1,37) = 4.80$, $p < .05$) for persons with type 2 diabetes. Furthermore, those with type 1 diabetes who see themselves as doers of their self-care behaviors were almost seven times more likely to have good diabetes control compared to those who are less likely to see themselves as doers of their diabetes self-care behaviors (χ^2 (1, N = 131) = 5.95, p = .01, Odd Ratio = 6.92).

Overall, researchers have determined that the SD-D is a reliable and valid measure of self-as-doer identity specific to diabetes self-care behaviors. Doer identification, as was originally conceptualized, can be modified and measured in a standardized form to represent self-care behavior management for a chronic disease. If diabetes-specific self-as-doer identities can be created into a standardized measure, then it also likely that the self-as-doer identity can be modified for other clinical populations with prescribed self-care management requirements. In addition to the utility of a standardized measure, it is also of value to note that again, the self-as-doer identity predicted self-care behaviors for a clinical population. The results of the study support the theoretical background of the self-as-doer identity in that seeing oneself as the doer of a behavior can promote behavioral engagement despite the behavior being unpleasant and unrewarding. For example, those with type 1 diabetes who saw themselves as doers of their diabetes self-care behaviors were more likely to adhere to a specific diabetes diet which included resisting sweets and limiting certain food groups. Moreover, that individuals with type 1 diabetes were almost seven times more likely to have good diabetes control if they had a higher doer identity specific to diabetes self-care management provides evidence for the power of doer identity in motivating behavior change in clinical populations.

What might have made the doer identity particularly salient for clinical populations is the illness identity that accompanies a diagnosis. For instance, chronic diseases such as diabetes, hypertension, or heart disease require a host of lifestyle changes in order to avoid serious health complications. To that end, the required self-care management serves as a day-to-day reminder of the disease and behaviors required to manage that disease. Furthermore, management of that disease is generally driven by a set of expectations and requirements from health care professions. These disease management behaviors are often quite rigid whereas individuals from non-clinical populations have more autonomy in deciding the type of health behaviors to engage in. The personal responsibility of self-care management, the explicit behaviors required for management, and the need for identification with the disease and its corresponding behaviors create a unique environment for the application of a doer identity. Because doer identity is about creating a self-concept related to behavior and doing a behavior rather than being rewarded for it, doer identification is likely to provide the motivation needed to engage and sustain health behavior changes for clinical populations. Although the research reviewed here is specific to those with diabetes, it is quite likely that doer identification, given its universal and diverse applicability, can be use among those with other chronic illnesses to promote health behavior change and maintenance. For example, encouraging an individual with heart disease to see themselves as a "daily walker" may provide the motivation needed to engage in those behaviors and to sustain them. Likewise, helping a client with HIV develop an identity as "medication taker" could promote the enactment of behavior beyond the experience of the negative side effects of taking that medication. Overall, the self-as-doer identity is particularly well suited to promote behaviors within clinical populations.

Having established that doer identification predicts self-care behaviors in a clinical population like diabetes and that the measurement of the construct can be standardized to represent disease-specific self-care behaviors, we would like to turn now to discussing how the self-as-doer fits in with existing psychological factors that affect self-care management in individuals with diabetes. Within the health behavior change literature, it is well documented that health behavior change and maintenance happen not on account of one variable alone, but when considering how variables work in relationship with one another (Riekert, Ockene, & Pbert, 2014). Programs theoretically grounded in health behavioral models which address the relationship among several variables have been more successful in creating and sustaining behavior change than programs not grounded in health behavior change models (Fishbein, 2002; Near & Zimmerman, 2005). As such, it is valuable to consider the role that self-a-doer identity might play in existing health models. If a self-as-doer identity has been found to increase health behaviors, then knowing how it works alongside of important agents of change like self-efficacy, for example, is likely to bolster the ability of researchers and interventionists to find ways to promote health behavior change among clinical populations. To address this need, Brouwer and Mosack (2012) explored the role that doer identification had between self-efficacy and self-care behaviors for those with diabetes.

Self-as-Doer for Diabetes and Self-Efficacy in Diabetes Self-Care Management

Self-efficacy, the perceived ability to successfully engage in a goal-directed behavior (Bandura, 1986, 1998), is a prominent and well-studied factor found to positively influence many behavior changes in clinical populations. Self-efficacy plays a vital role in health behavior change (Bandura, 2004), and numerous health behaviors have been increased through interventions focused on self-efficacy (Higgins, Middleton, Winner, & Janelle, 2014; Holmes, Hughes, & Morrison, 2014; Sarkar, Fisher, & Schillinger, 2006; Sheeran et al., 2016). However, the mechanisms by which self-efficacy create change are less well understood, especially as it relates to identity. Given that self-efficacy is the perceived ability to perform a behavior, it may be that identity, especially in the form of seeing oneself as the doer of one's behavior, could play a vital role in explaining how ability leads to behavior change. For example, consider an individual who has heart disease and is attempting to become more physically active. The degree to which he believes that he can go out on a walk every morning will certainly affect whether he actually does go out on a walk. Yet knowing that he has the ability to walk (e.g., he has walking shoes, has the time, and can walk without pain), does not guarantee that he will go walking every morning. There may be external barriers (e.g., it is raining outside, his muscles are sore) or his motivation may be low. Now consider the role that a self-as-doer identity might play in the relationship between self-efficacy and behavioral enactment. According to the self-as-doer theory, having an identity as a "walker" in this example would increase motivation to engage in the behavior and cause the individual to walk despite the barriers. Thus if it were raining outside, the individual, having a doer identity as a "walker," would be motivated to find another way to fulfill that identity by perhaps going to the gym or walking on a treadmill. Having a doer identity would then lead the individual to be more likely to walk than if the decision were based on ability alone (e.g., I can walk, but it's raining outside today, so I will not walk today). As such, perhaps the ability to do a behavior can enhance one's doer identity, which consequently leads to more successful behavior change.

To test this idea, Brouwer and Mosack (2012) asked the same adults with diabetes to complete questions about diabetes-specific self-efficacy, diabetes self-care behaviors, and the SD-D. Self-as-doer identity, as measured by the SD-D, was proposed to be a mediating variable in the relationship between self-efficacy and diabetes self-care behaviors. That is, it was expected that as self-efficacy increased, so did self-as-doer identity which consequently increased self-care behaviors (see conceptual model in Figure 5.1).

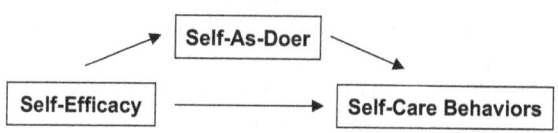

Figure 5.1 A conceptual model of the intervening effects of the self-as-doer on the relationship between self-efficacy and self-care behaviors

Source: From " 'I am a blood sugar checker': Intervening effects of the self-as-doer identity on the relationship between self-efficacy and diabetes self-care behaviors" by A. M. Brouwer and K. E. Mosack, 2012, *Self and Identity*, *11*, p. 479. Copyright [2012] by Psychology Press. Adapted with permission.

The researchers found that for people with type 1 diabetes, self-as-doer identity was an important factor that explained how self-efficacy affected exercise, diet, blood glucose monitoring, foot care, and medication taking self-care behaviors. For people with type 2 diabetes, self-as-doer was a significant mediator between self-efficacy and diet, blood glucose monitoring, and exercise, but not for foot care or medication taking self-care behaviors (see Brouwer & Mosack, 2012 for study design and statistical details). Findings suggested, as expected, that as the ability for a behavior increased so did one's identity as the doer of that behavior. This then led to the increase of the behavior. For some self-care behaviors (exercise, blood glucose monitoring, and foot care for those with type 1 diabetes and exercise and blood glucose monitoring for those with type 2 diabetes), self-as-doer identity explained the entire relationship between self-efficacy and the behavior, thereby further supporting the claim that the effect of ability to do a behavior on a corresponding behavior is facilitated by seeing oneself as the doer of that behavior.

Overall, the study further supports the theoretical role of the self-as-doer identity in existing health models. It suggests that doer identification can be used to bolster existing attempts for behavior change. For example, if a clinical intervention is attempting to increase adherence for medication taking behaviors and has focused on improving individuals' self-efficacy for that behavior, interventionists could increase the likelihood of its success by also addressing the degree to which one see themselves as a "medication taker." Incorporating exercises to enhance doer identity is likely to enhance the desired behavior. Many behavior change programs for clinical populations have self-efficacy elements built into them. Adding exercises to address or promote a self-as-doer identity could be easily incorporated and generalized to other clinical populations.

Conclusion

Just as the self-as-doer identity works well with non-clinical populations, doer identification can also be easily incorporated into health promotion efforts for clinical populations. Indeed, doer identity played a unique role in predicting diabetes self-care behaviors and in explaining how self-efficacy affects diabetes self-care behaviors. Furthermore, the research reviewed established that doer identification can be measured and used to predict diabetes self-care management via a standardized measure. Although the evidence reviewed was for clinical populations with diabetes, the application of any of these findings is relevant for other clinical populations. Much of self-care management for individuals with diabetes can be generalized to self-care behaviors required in other chronic illnesses (e.g., eating a healthy diet, getting regular physical activity, taking medications, etc.). If thinking about oneself as a "healthy eater" can increase the likelihood that an individual with diabetes will eat more healthily because it is part of their disease management, then it is also likely that a "healthy eater" self-as-doer identity can promote healthy eating behaviors for individuals with cardiovascular disease, for example. How the self-as-doer identity can be used to promote health behavior change and maintenance in other populations, both clinical and non-clinical, will be the topic of the next and final chapter.

Appendix 5.1

Self-as-Doer-Diabetes Measure[1]

Self-as-Doer-Diabetes

Instructions: *Below are some statements that people with diabetes have used to describe themselves in relation to their diabetes goals and self-care behaviors. Using the scale below, please indicate how well these phrases describe or fit you by circling the number next to each phrase. Remember—there are **no right or wrong** answers.*

	Does Not Describe Me Well At All	Does Not Describe Me Well	Neutral	Describes Me Well	Describes Me Very Well
	1	2	3	4	5

To what degree do you see yourself as a . . . .

1. Sweets Resister	1	2	3	4	5
2. Blood Sugar Controller	1	2	3	4	5
3. Diabetes Social Support Receiver	1	2	3	4	5
4. Fruit Eater	1	2	3	4	5
5. High Blood Sugar Avoider	1	2	3	4	5
6. Consistent Blood Sugar Record Keeper	1	2	3	4	5
7. Diabetes Research Supporter	1	2	3	4	5
8. Daily Activity Doer	1	2	3	4	5
9. Medication/Insulin Adjuster	1	2	3	4	5

	Does Not Describe Me Well At All	Does Not Describe Me Well	Neutral	Describes Me Well	Describes Me Very Well
	1	2	3	4	5
10. Diabetes Social Support Seeker	1	2	3	4	5
11. Frequent Blood Glucose Checker	1	2	3	4	5
12. Diabetes Treatment Follower	1	2	3	4	5
13. Daily Activity Balancer	1	2	3	4	5
14. Diabetes Teacher	1	2	3	4	5
15. Cholesterol Monitor	1	2	3	4	5
16. Frequent Eye Checker	1	2	3	4	5
17. Regular Diabetes Doctor Appointment Attender	1	2	3	4	5
18. Good Hemoglobin A1c Getter	1	2	3	4	5
19. Strenuous Exerciser	1	2	3	4	5
20. Punctual Medication/ Insulin Taker	1	2	3	4	5
21. Family Support Receiver	1	2	3	4	5
22. Daily Fat Limiter	1	2	3	4	5
23. Diabetes Information Gatherer	1	2	3	4	5
24. Frequent Exerciser	1	2	3	4	5
25. Blood Pressure Checker	1	2	3	4	5
26. Diabetes Treatment Collaborator	1	2	3	4	5
27. Healthy Eater	1	2	3	4	5
28. Relaxer	1	2	3	4	5
29. Moderate Exerciser	1	2	3	4	5

(*Continued*)

(*Continued*)

	Does Not Describe Me Well At All	Does Not Describe Me Well	Neutral	Describes Me Well	Describes Me Very Well
	1	2	3	4	5
30. Correct Medication/ Insulin Dose Taker	1	2	3	4	5
31. Diabetes Health Care Team Support Receiver	1	2	3	4	5
32. Frequent Foot Checker	1	2	3	4	5
33. Stress Controller	1	2	3	4	5
34. Medication/Insulin Taker	1	2	3	4	5
35. Diabetes Diet Follower	1	2⸴	3	4	5
36. Diabetes Health Care Team Communicator	1	2	3	4	5
37. Diabetes Events Participator	1	2	3	4	5
38. Vegetable Eater	1	2	3	4	5
39. Complications Preventer	1	2	3	4	5
40. Stress Preventer	1	2	3	4	5
41. Anaerobic Exerciser (short—ex: weight lifting)	1	2	3	4	5
42. Overall Body Caretaker	1	2	3	4	5

Note

1. From "Self-as-Doer for diabetes: Development and validation of a diabetes-specific measure of doer identification" by A. M. Brouwer and K. E. Mosack, 2013, *Journal of Nursing Measurement, 21*, pp. 208–209. Copyright [2013] by Springer Publishing Company, LLC. Reprinted with permission.

References

American Diabetes Association (2016). Standards of medical care in diabetes—2016. *Diabetes Care, 39*(1, Suppl.), S1–S12.

Bandura, A. (1986). *Social foundations of thought and action: A social cognitive theory.* Englewood Cliffs, NJ: Prentice Hall.

Bandura, A. (1998). Health promotion from the perspective of social cognitive theory. *Psychology and Health, 13*, 623–649.

Bandura, A. (2004). Health promotion by social cognitive means. *Health Education & Behavior, 31*, 143–164. doi: 10.1177/1090198104263660

Brouwer, A. M. (2008, May). *Predictors of self-care behaviors: Self-efficacy and self-as-doer.* Poster presented at the Midwestern Psychological Association Conference in Chicago, IL.

Brouwer, A. M., & Mosack, K. E. (2012). "I am a blood sugar checker": Intervening effects of the self-as-doer identity on the relationship between self-efficacy and diabetes self-care behaviors. *Self and Identity, 11*, 472–491. doi: 10.1080/15298868.2011.603901

Brouwer, A. M., & Mosack, K. E. (2013). Self-as-doer for diabetes: Development and validation of a diabetes-specific measure of doer identification. *Journal of Nursing Measurement, 21*, 188–209. doi: 10.1891/1061-3749.21.2.188

Crutzen, R., Viechtbauer, W., Spigt, M., & Kotz, D. (2015). Differential attrition in health behaviour change trials: A systematic review and meta-analysis. *Psychology & Health, 30*(1), 122–134. doi: 10.1080/08870446.2014.953526

de Bruin, M., McCambridge, J., & Prins, J. M. (2015). Reducing the risk of bias in health behaviour change trials: Improving trial design, reporting, or bias assessment criteria? A review and case study. *Psychology & Health, 30*(1), 8–34. doi: 10.1080/08870446.2014.953531

Dumville, J. C., Torgerson, D. J., & Hewitt, C. E. (2006). Reporting attrition in randomised controlled trials. *British Medical Journal, 332*, 969. doi: 10.1136/bmj.332.7547.969

Elliot, A. J. (2006). The hierarchical model of approach-avoidance motivation. *Motivation and Emotion, 30*, 111–116, doi: 10.1007/s11031-006-9028-7

Fishbein, M. (2002). The role of theory in HIV prevention. In D. F. Marks (Ed.), *The health psychology reader* (pp. 120–126). London: Sage.

Higgins, T. J., Middleton, K. R., Winner, L., & Janelle, C. M. (2014). Physical activity interventions differentially affect exercise task and barrier self-efficacy: A meta-analysis. *Health Psychology, 33*(8), 891–903. doi: 10.1037/a0033864

Holmes, E. F., Hughes, D. A., & Morrison, V. L. (2014). Predicting adherence to medications using health psychology theories: A systematic review of 20 years of empirical research. *Value in Health, 17*(8), 863–876. doi: 10.1016/j. jval.2014.08.2671

Near, S. M., & Zimmerman, R. S. (2005). Health behavior theory and cumulative knowledge regarding health behaviors: Are we moving in the right direction? *Health Education Research, 20,* 275–290. doi: 10.1093/her/cyg113

Riekert, K. A., Ockene, J. K., & Pbert, L. (Eds.). (2014). *The handbook of health behavior change.* New York: Springer Publishing.

Sarkar, U., Fisher, L., & Schillinger, D. (2006). Is self-efficacy associated with diabetes self-management across race/ethnicity and health literacy? *Diabetes Care, 29,* 823–829. doi: 10.2337/diacare.29.04.06.dc05–1615

Sheeran, P., Maki, A., Montanaro, E., Avishai-Yitshak, A., Bryan, A., Klein, W. P., . . . Rothman, A. J. (2016). The impact of changing attitudes, norms, and self-efficacy on health-related intentions and behavior: A meta-analysis. *Health Psychology, 35*(11), 1178–1188. doi: 10.1037/hea0000387

Shirvastava, S. R., Shrivastava, P. S., & Ramasamy, J. (2013). Role of self-care in management of diabetes mellitus. *Journal of Diabetes & Metabolic Disorders, 12,* 1–5. doi: 10.1186/2251-6581-12-14

Taylor, S. E. (2013). Social cognition and health. In D. E. Carlston (Ed.), *The Oxford handbook of social cognition* (pp. 876–893). New York: Oxford University Press.

Williams, S. L., Haskard-Zolnierek, K. B., & Dimatteo, M. R. (2014). Psychosocial predictors of behavior change. In K. A. Riekert, J. K. Ockene, & L. Pbert (Eds.), *The handbook of health behavior change* (4th ed., pp. 69–86). New York: Springer.

6 Recommendations for Using the Self-as-Doer Identity

Amanda M. Brouwer and Katie E. Mosack

The self-as-doer identity, an identity that describes one as the doer of his or her behavior, is a unique and accessible motivational identity which can be easily incorporated into health behavior change efforts. As introduced in Chapter 2, the self-as-doer identity is rooted in identity theory, which suggests that identity develops as a result of social roles which supply meaning and purpose. Doer identification has been argued to be unique in that the act of calling oneself a doer (e.g., a "runner" or "healthy eater") creates motivation to go beyond other factors to facilitate health behavior change. Examples of how the doer identity is developed in clinical (e.g., people living with diabetes) and non-clinical (e.g., people interested in achieving a healthy diet or regularly engaging in physical activity) populations provides a framework on how the doer identity is created and conceptualized. Measurement of the doer identity, both in its original and customized form, further capitalizes on the diverse ways in which the self-as-doer can be used. Furthermore, the results reviewed from research in both clinical and non-clinical populations demonstrate the power of the self-as-doer in promoting health behavior change and maintenance in multiple populations.

Research on the self-as-doer supports arguments proposed by identity theorists (Biddle et al., 1985; Stryker & Burke, 2000) that identity is a socially constructed motivation wherein individuals behave in ways that are consistent with their sense of self. As such, focusing on the self-as-doer identity, that is, helping individuals see themselves as the doer of their behaviors, can be relevant in both clinical and research settings in which there is a focus on health behavior change. Moreover, the flexible nature of the self-as-doer identity enables its application in relation to a wide range of behaviors (e.g., increased physical activity, reduced tobacco intake, improved sleep habits, improved medication adherence, etc.). What follows is a discussion of how the self-as-doer can be applied to various clinical and non-clinical populations, how it can be used in both clinical and research settings, its limitations, and our suggestions for future work within these settings.

Self-as-Doer in Various Populations

Researchers have made a clear case for using the self-as-doer within specific populations seeking to make health behavior changes. Current evidence demonstrates that the self-as-doer can be used to predict self-care behaviors in a clinical population (e.g., among patients living with diabetes) as well as physical activity and healthy eating behaviors in non-clinical populations (Brouwer, n.d.; Brouwer & Mosack, 2015). The ability to connect identity and behavior to provide an additional source of motivation to encourage both the instigation and maintenance of behavior change is what makes the self-as-doer unique and accessible for use in multiple populations. That is, the self-as-doer has the potential to be used within any population that is seeking to make health behavior changes that require persistence and motivation to enact and maintain. Therefore, its use could be widespread. For instance, it could be used among clinical populations of people who are asked to follow specific disease-management regimens (e.g., cardiovascular disease, obesity, hypertension, HIV, etc.) or among individuals outside of the clinical context who are attempting to make various health behavior changes such as increasing physical activity, reducing tobacco intake, improving sleeping habits, and reducing stress.

The unique attributes of the self-as-doer (see Chapter 2) are what make it applicable to a variety of populations. The self-as-doer can be either domain-specific or general (see Chapter 2). As such, it could be used to assess a wide array of prescribed health behaviors within a health-care context (e.g., medication use, restrictions in diet, disease-specific regimens, etc.) or behaviors that are universally relevant (e.g., sleeping habits, tobacco use, physical activity, etc.). Furthermore, researchers have demonstrated that the self-as-doer identity can be accessed even for those who do not already consider themselves as the "doer" of their behaviors (Houser-Marko & Sheldon, 2006). The implication of this finding for clinical populations is that the self-as-doer identity can be relevant whether one is facing a new chronic disease diagnosis or whether one has been living with an illness for some time and has had time to develop a disease-related identity. Likewise, for non-clinical populations, the easy accessibility of the doer identity suggests that it can be developed for health behaviors that have yet to be internalized as important to health behavior change.

Self-as-Doer as an Assessment Tool

The self-as-doer has a number of potential uses in the context of clinical practice and research. One specific use is that of an assessment or screening tool to measure the existing degree of one's doer identity. In both clinical and research settings, the tool can be used to assess both baseline doer identity and how the self-as-doer identity changes over the course of an intervention or behavior change session. Having such a tool would help the clinician to develop a plan for behavior change. For example, assessing self-as-doer identity at the beginning of a program would give insight on existing doer identity in such a way that clinicians can develop or modify health behavior change programs to address lack of motivation or identity associated with the expected behavior change. Modifications could enhance motivation or identity associated with expected behaviors and consequently bolster the outcomes of the behavior change program. Additionally, the evaluation of the degree to which a patient identifies him or herself as the doer of his or her behavior could also be used to individualize subsequent interventions or program plans. Within research settings, both baseline and subsequent self-as-doer scores can be compared with other variables of interest (e.g., health behavior locus of control) to get a better sense of the degree to which the self-as-doer is implicated in health behavior change.

Since the self-as-doer can be easily customized for different populations (see Chapters 4 and 5 for examples), the self-as-doer identity instrument could be modified to address self-as-doer identities specific to any targeted health behaviors of interest. For example, consider a researcher who is interested in exploring how a doer identity related to medication adherence might affect the degree to which patients with hypertension take their medications. In this example, the researcher could tailor the generic self-as-doer measure in a way that asks participants to create goals (and subsequent doer identities) specifically related to medication adherence (see Appendix 6.1 for an example). One could then use the measure as a way to assess how a medication adherence-related doer identity changes throughout the course of an adherence intervention. Notably, the self-as-doer measure is relatively short and simple, which limits the burden placed on the patient to complete it during a standard clinical appointment.

Given the potential to assess self-as-doer identity for specific populations, one avenue of future research with the self-as-doer identity is to identify a population for which there are a specific set of requisite health behaviors and to develop self-as-doer identities specific to those behaviors that could then be generalized across all patients with such a condition. In doing so, one could then create a standardized measure of self-as-doer identity for this population. (See Chapter 5 for examples of how this is done for individuals with diabetes.) For example, if one were to apply the self-as-doer identity to a population of individuals with cardiovascular disease, there are commonly prescribed health behavior change recommendations for this population such as following a healthy diet (e.g., eating more fruits, vegetable, whole grains, etc.), reducing sodium, becoming more physically active, reducing stress (e.g., through meditation or practicing yoga), learning to relax, and taking prescribed medications (National Institutes of Health, 2014). In much the same way as the self-as-doer identity measure has been custom- ized for individuals with diabetes (see Brouwer & Mosack, 2013), one could identify goals related to heart disease management and create corresponding doer identities which could be used to develop and validate a standardized measure of self-as-doer identity for patients with cardiovascular disease. (See Chapter 3 for the process of creating doer identities.) For example, if requisite behaviors for managing cardiovascular disease included reduc- ing sodium in one's diet or taking prescribed medications, then the doer identities of "sodium reducer" and "medication taker" could be added to a customized measure of doer identity for those with cardiovascular disease. Once measured to be reliable and valid, this tool could then be used in both clinical and research settings to asses self-as-doer identity specific to car- diovascular disease management.

Self-as-Doer as an Educational Tool

The self-as-doer measure can also be used as an educational tool in that it teaches individuals new ways of thinking about behavior change and how to become motivated to do so. The self-as-doer measure provides an active learning resource for health care professionals in that it engages the patient by requiring the patient to create goals and subsequent doer identities and then to discuss how these doer identities might be helpful in achieving health behavior change. The process of creating health behavior-specific goals and translating those goals into statements which describe the indi- vidual as the doer of his or her behavior is a cognitive task which has potential to spur thoughts and subsequent behaviors about needed behavior change. Furthermore, the self-as-doer task gives individuals an opportunity to discuss their current behaviors and how one could go about modifying them in a way to achieve their desired goals. Overall, thinking about one- self as the doer of one's behavioral objectives provides a resource (i.e., a doer identity to identify with when deciding how to change behavior) for the individual to begin making subsequent behavior changes. As such, the self-as-doer measure can serve as an educational resource for those looking for a process to assist patients in thinking about their approach to behavior change.

One way to use the self-as-doer as an educational tool may be for diabetes educators or other health professionals working with a population of indi- viduals living with diabetes. These health care professionals might consider having patients complete the self-as-doer measure as a way to generate con- versation about diabetes-specific health behavior goals and specific ways, via doer identity, to meet those goals. As an example, consider the following scenario.

> Dr. Shoma, who works with individuals who have diabetes, has a patient, Candace, who is struggling to enact certain diabetes self-care management behaviors. In a session with Candace, Dr. Shoma presents the self-as-doer measure to Candace and asks her to create 3 or 4 goals related to her diabetes self-care management. Candace identifies that she would like to "check her blood sugar more frequently," "eat more fruits and vegetables," and "take her medications regularly." Dr. Shoma then reviews the steps (see Chapter 3) for creating self-as-doer identities from these goals. Candace creates the self-as-doer goals of "frequent blood sugar checker," "fruit and vegetable eater," and "regular medication taker." Dr. Shoma then assists Candace with the final step of the measure and asks Candace to rate herself on a scale of 1 (does not describe me well at all) to 5 (describes me very well) as to how well each of the doer identity phrases describes her currently. After Candace's evaluation, Dr. Shoma asks Candace to describe what her created doer identities represent to her. That is, Dr. Shoma asks questions such as, "What does a frequent blood sugar checker look like to you?" "How would you describe a frequent blood sugar checker?" and "What does a frequent blood sugar checker do?" Dr. Shoma then helps Candace find ways to conceptualize herself as a "frequent blood sugar checker" or "fruit and vegetable eater" to a greater degree than she indicated on the evaluation. Dr. Shoma asks questions such as, "What would it take for you to see yourself as a frequent blood sugar checker to a greater degree than you do right now?" Together they brainstorm ways to develop this identity more fully and overcome potential barriers to developing the identity.

Such an educational tool could be used outside clinical populations as well. Consider, for example, a weight loss management program. Creating weight loss goals and subsequent doer identities related to weight loss could introduce those in the program to new ways of thinking about achieving their weight loss goals. Rather than, for example, only having the target goal of losing a certain amount of weight (which is often a consequence of other distinct behaviors), discussing the self-as-doer might promote the development of other identities to ascribe to which are more discrete in nature and may promote greater behavioral change. Being a "weight loser," for example, might require that one increase their physical activity behaviors. Creating and identifying with a self-as-doer identity such as a "weekly exerciser" would give the individual a specific behavior to focus on in the pursuit of losing weight. In the same vein, the use of the self-as-doer in this context could also help a person not just lose weight but maintain the weight through modified health behaviors. For example, eating a healthy diet is one way to lose weight, but is also necessary for long-term weight maintenance. Thus seeing oneself as a "fruit eater" or "vegetable eater" instead of only a "weight loser" could create diverse identities which promote distinct behaviors that help individuals not only achieve their weight loss goals, but also help them achieve weight maintenance.

To further enhance the degree to which the self-as-doer can be used as an educational tool to elicit health behavior change and to facilitate participant buy-in, the self-as-doer instrument and intervention could be used in conjunction with existing health behavior change approaches such as motivational interviewing (Miller & Rollnick, 2002). Motivational interviewing is an intervention approach focused on helping individuals become more aware of their motivations and skills for change and empowering individuals to take responsibility for their own behaviors (for more information on motivational interviewing see Miller & Rollnick, 2002). Motivational interviewing is also designed to help patients who are ambivalent or reluctant to change their behaviors identify the benefits and disadvantages of behavior change. In short, motivational interviewing assists individuals in developing the motivation to make positive behavioral changes to achieve their health behavior goals. Since one of the objectives of motivational interviewing is to help individuals identify their motivations and ways to take responsibility for behavioral change, the self-as-doer task could serve as a mechanism for identifying motivations through the development of goals for behavior change and how then to take individual responsibility for those behaviors by thinking about how one can see oneself as the doer of those behaviors. For instance, the self-as-doer measure could be completed before a counseling session and used as a foundation to help elicit patients' motivations for behavior change and ideas for possible impediments to that change. Created self-as-doer identities could serve as a tool for discussing individualized identities for behavioral goals. Another core tenant of motivational interviewing is autonomy, giving the patient responsibility and respecting their decision-making abilities. The self-as-doer promotes autonomy in that creating goals and doer identities are a mechanism for an individual to personalize his or her health behavior-related identities. That the individual can take responsibility for the creation of doer identities has potential to empower the individual in his or her desire for behavior change. This empowerment is an important component of motivational interviewing and further demonstrates how self-as-doer identity can complement motivational interviewing.

Self-as-Doer as an Intervention

Using the self-as-doer identity as a stand-alone intervention or to supplement an existing intervention has the potential to elicit new health behavior change and to encourage the maintenance of health behavior change. As described in Chapter 4, the self-as-doer intervention led to the maintenance of healthy eating behavior among those who received it whereas others who did not receive the intervention actually decreased their overall healthy eating behaviors over time. The intervention is easy to incorporate as it requires minimal training and resources and the time it takes to complete the intervention is relatively short. Given the simplicity of the intervention, participants have little trouble completing it and the intervention task resonates well with most participants. In fact, in our experience (Brouwer & Mosack, 2015), some participants even went above and beyond the expectations of the intervention by writing doer phrases in their personal food diaries and sharing behavior changes with the researcher, referencing the doer phrases in their conversations about such changes. This intervention could be easily modified for other populations or incorporated into an education session or any health behavior change intervention in clinical or research contexts. For example, in a self-as-doer intervention designed to assist individuals in modifying their health behaviors to reduce cardiovascular disease, those at risk could identify goals related to the needed health behavior modifications (e.g., diet modifications, stress reduction, medication adherence) and subsequently develop self-as-doer identity statements to describe the doer of each created goal. Clinicians or researchers could then deliver the intervention as described in Chapter 4. Because the common thread among diverse populations in need of better health is the motivation to engage in and maintain health behavior change and that the self-as-doer identity intervention is designed to provide a source of motivation for that behavior change and maintenance, the intervention can be used quite broadly.

The self-as-doer identity intervention could also be added to existing programs as another tool to boost efficacy within in a program or intervention. For example, in a 12-week weight management program the self-as-doer identity could be added as a topic for one of the weekly session. Given that the intervention does not require an extensive amount of time to complete (approximately 30–45 minutes), participants could complete it within one session. The intervention could also be modified so that small groups of individuals could receive the intervention together, rather than in a one-to-one session as was done in the initial study. For example, self-as-doer measure forms could be handed out to group members and they could collectively be instructed to complete the first part of the task by creating 6–8 goals related to their health behavior change. The clinician could monitor each individual as they create goals and offer suggestions to ensure the goals are specific to the desired behavioral outcomes. Then the clinician could provide the group with instructions for the second phase of the intervention, creating doer identity statements. Again, as participants individually work through this phase, the clinician could monitor doer identity development and provide feedback as needed. Furthermore, the group members could help each other develop doer phrases by sharing their ideas and brainstorming about various alternatives to achieve better health outcomes. Following this same procedure, participants could then rate how much each doer phrase currently described them. For the final phase of the intervention, reflecting on how doer identities are or are not consistent with one's self-concept, group members could get in pairs and share their responses to a series of questions asked by the clinician with one another. The clinician would ask the group to identify a doer identity that they, individually, rated low (i.e., below 3), and then say in accordance with the intervention protocol, "Picture yourself as that identity. What would that look like?" After a brief moment to allow participants to think about their individual identities, the clinician or researcher could then say, "Now share your thoughts about this question with your partner." The remaining questions in the interview could be followed using a similar procedure. It is important to note that although it is likely that the intervention administered in a group setting would have a similar impact for individuals as in a one-to-one setting, the evidence for the self-as-doer intervention in behavior maintenance has only been evaluated in one-on-one conditions. However, the primary function of the intervention (i.e., getting participants to think about doer identities and how they can see themselves as that identity to a greater degree) is still likely to be achieved whether done in a group or in an individual setting.

Limitations and Recommendations for Improvement

Although preliminary research on the self-as-doer identity has shown promise for its research and clinical utility in promoting health behavior change and maintenance, there are certainly limitations that must be acknowledged and recommendations for improvement for its use within both research and clinical contexts. As an assessment and measurement tool, the self-as-doer has been used successfully to predict future behavior. It is important, however, to assess both past and current behaviors in order to prevent the prediction from becoming circular. That is, when asking individuals to create behavioral goals and doer statements from such goals, one could be asking individuals to indicate whether they are currently acting to attain those goals, and in doing so may be measuring current behaviors, rather than the intended self-as-doer identity. Current behaviors rather than the self-as-doer identity then would become the predictor of future behaviors. Second, in order to draw conclusions about the degree to which the doer intervention is responsible for change, researchers should randomize individuals to one of two different conditions, the only difference of which would be the inclusion of the doer intervention. Of course, within the realm of individual behavior change objectives (e.g., in clinical practice), an experimental or quasi-experimental structure is simply not feasible. However, even in the clinical context, we recommend measuring behavior at regular intervals during the intervention (depending on how long the engagement lasts), at the end of the intervention, and, if possible, at regular time points after the intervention in order to empirically evaluate whether and at what rate behavior change has occurred.

Although it is not possible to isolate the effects of the self-as-doer to explain health behavior change outside of the realm of an experiment, we have found that the self-as-doer has contributed to behavior change independent of other relevant factors in the series of studies that we have conducted in our research labs. For example, the self-as-doer identity has been found to predict diabetes self-care behaviors, especially for those with type 1 diabetes, above and beyond self-efficacy, locus of control, self-determinism, and other psycho-social constructs related to diabetes self-care management (Brouwer & Mosack, 2013). Likewise, the self-as-doer predicted physical activity behaviors among young adults beyond existing motivational beliefs such as self-determinism, exercise motivations, exercise identity, and self-efficacy (Brouwer, n.d.). Finally, in an intervention designed to explore the causal effects of the self-as-doer identity on healthy diet change, those who received the self-as-doer intervention had significantly higher healthy eating behaviors than those who did not receive the intervention 1 month after the intervention was administered (Brouwer & Mosack, 2015).

Although findings from several studies support the use of the self-as-doer construct in creating behavior change across contexts, there are several ways in which it could be improved. In our initial diet experiment, the self-as-doer was only introduced once and not again mentioned at follow-up appointments (Brouwer & Mosack, 2015). Although the self-as-doer intervention demonstrated promise for behavior maintenance with respect to diet-related behaviors because it predicted the maintenance of existing healthy eating behaviors, it did not demonstrate an increase in novel healthy eating behaviors. In hindsight, outcomes might have been improved had we included a booster session to the self-as-doer intervention in order to enhance the saliency of a self-as-doer identity. Booster sessions are additional sessions that occur after the intervention and are designed to remind or reinforce the active component of the intervention. Therefore, reminding participants about their generated self-as-doer identities or engaging in a discussion about what they are doing to identify with those identities may have elicited motivation to expand new healthy behaviors in addition to maintaining existing ones. Booster sessions have, in fact, been found to create greater maintenance of health behaviors such as exercise (Fjeldsoe, Neuhaus, Winkler, & Eakin, 2011; Fleig, Pomp, Schwarzer, & Lippke, 2013; Jancey et al., 2011) and smoking cessation (Metz et al., 2007) compared to those who did not receive the booster sessions. Given the evidence for the effectiveness of booster sessions in other related behavior change interventions, it is likely that such an enhancement to the current intervention would improve participant behavioral outcomes.

Another recommendation to bolster the effect of the self-as-doer intervention would be to add supplemental identity enhancing activities that would more strongly foster doer identification. Identity theorists posit that meaning and purpose are developed out of social roles and that the greater identification one has with that social role, the more one will come to behave in accordance with that role (Burke, 1991; Stryker & Burke, 2000). As such, providing opportunities for individuals to develop greater meaning associated with their doer identities might enhance the degree to which they identify with them and may consequently lead to greater behavior change. When developing the self-as-doer identity, Houser-Marko and Sheldon (2006) conducted a study to determine whether they could elicit doer identity. They had participants read a motivational story (i.e., *The Little Engine That Could*) and apply the moral of the story to themselves. They found that those who applied the motivational moral to themselves in an essay persisted for longer at a physical activity task than did those who applied the moral to another person or did not read a motivational story. As such, one might add a journaling component to the intervention where participants are asked not just to verbally identify how they see themselves as a doer and what they can do to be more like that identity, but to write an essay on how that identity could be applied to themselves and consequently aid them in their pursuits of behavior change and overcoming barriers to achieving their behavior change goals. One might also encourage participants to create reminders of their identity in places they frequent as a way to visibly represent their identity to themselves and to others, and thereby identify with their doer identities to a greater degree. For example, if a participant's identity was to become a "water drinker," perhaps asking that participant to put a water bottle on his kitchen counter to remind him of his identity might be a way to boost that identity. Another way to promote a doer identity through outward projections of the identity would be to encourage participants or patients to find ways to talk about their identity with others, whether that be through posting on social media (e.g., "Today I am a veggie eater" with a corresponding picture of the individual eating a salad) or in conversations with friends (e.g., "Sorry, I'm going to pass on the dessert tonight, I'm trying to be a healthy eater"). Consistent with identity theory, the more one outwardly portrays the identity, the greater the need to act in accordance with that identity. As such, these environmental reminders (e.g., a water bottle for the "water drinker") and conversations about one's doer identity with others have potential to boost and maintain that identity in a way that is likely to promote corresponding behavior and strengthen the impact of the self-as-doer intervention.

Self-as-Doer and Health Behavior Maintenance

One of the strengths of the self-as-doer doer identity, as supported by foundational research, is that it has potential, in various contexts, to facilitate the maintenance of health behavior changes. As discussed in earlier chapters, health behavior change is difficult and maintenance of that change proves even more challenging (Prapavessis et al., 2016; Spohr et al., 2015). Some might argue that motivation for initial change is relatively strong, but over time motivation to persist in those behaviors wanes. That the self-as-doer is an identity which aims not only to describe the individual in terms of a behavior, but that the behavioral identity provides motivation particularly in times when other environmental contexts are not reinforcing suggests that it is a vital construct to use to promote maintenance. That is, being able to call oneself a "healthy eater," "runner," or "medication taker" is what is providing the motivation to enact the behaviors to make such claims true. Although we suspect that the self-as-doer could be useful in interventions designed to maintain health behavior changes, research about prospective behavior change maintenance has yet to be conducted.

How the self-as-doer identity contributes to health behavior change maintenance has been discussed throughout the book. There are, however, additional ideas to consider when evaluating the effects of the self-as-doer on health behavior change that warrant further discussion here. The self-as-doer identity can be used over time to improve maintenance by providing reminders about the importance of that doer identity for the individuals. In accordance with identity theory, if individuals truly find meaning and purpose in the identities they create, then they will be motivated to behave in ways that help maintain that identity. Since the self-as-doer identity connects identity with behavior, then helping individuals to re-access the link between that self-concept and behavior may provide the additional motivation needed to maintain the behavior well after the initial change has been made. Ways to achieve this may be to ask participants regularly to evaluate how closely they feel they are a "healthy eater" in a specified period of time (e.g., a week). Additionally, if the self-as-doer identity intervention was used as a tool in an existing program (e.g., 12-week weight loss program), providing a booster session where participants were reminded about their doer identities could help with maintenance of their behaviors. Participants might even be asked to re-conceptualize their doer identities and discuss their progress in identifying with them to a stronger degree. One might also consider capitalizing on cognitive dissonance in that through various exercises individuals are made aware of the discrepancies between their current identities and their desired doer identities. The knowledge of the inconsistency might then motivate them to continue to engage in behaviors to achieve their desired self-as-doer identity.

Conclusion

In sum, the self-as-doer identity intervention has potential to be used in a variety of research and clinical settings with both clinical and non-clinical populations. A self-as-doer identity, which enables people to view themselves as the doer of their behaviors, plays an important role in not just the creation of health behavior changes but also the maintenance of those behaviors. We have described how the self-as-doer identity can be used as an assessment, educational, and intervention tool. Its use as an assessment tool can assist researchers and clinicians in measuring the degree of doer identity before or after health behavior interventions or health sessions. As an educational tool, the self-as-doer can provide interventionists with the opportunity to assist research participants and patients in developing strategies to both begin and maintain desired health behavior changes. Moreover, the use of the self-as-doer as a stand-alone intervention or in conjunction with other existing programs has potential to affect both short-term and long-term health behavior changes. Amid the sea of complicated and expensive approaches for improving overall health and reducing risks of disease, the self-as-doer identity offers a novel, forthright approach to assist researchers, clinicians, and those seeking to make meaningful, lasting health behavior changes.

References

Biddle, B. J., Bank, B. J., Anderson, D. S., Hauge, R., Keats, D. M., Keats, J. A., . . . Valantin, S. (1985). Social influence, self-referent identity labels and behavior. *The Sociological Quarterly, 26*, 159–185. doi: 10.1111/j.1533–8525.1985.tb00221.x

Brouwer, A. M. (n.d.). *Predicting physical activity with identity: The self-as-doer identity.* Unpublished manuscript.

Brouwer, A. M., & Mosack, K. E. (2013). Self-as-doer for diabetes: Development and validation of a diabetes-specific measure of doer identification. *Journal of Nursing Measurement, 21,* 188–209. doi: 10.1891/1061-3749.21.2.188

Brouwer, A. M., & Mosack, K. E. (2015). Motivating health diet behaviors: The self-as-doer identity. *Self and Identity, 14,* 638–653. doi: 10.1080/15298868.2015.1043335

Burke, P. J. (1991). An identity theory approach to commitment. *Social Psychology Quarterly, 54,* 239–251. Retrieved from www.jstor.org/stable/2786653

Fjeldsoe, B., Neuhaus, M., Winkler, E., & Eakin, E. (2011). Systematic review of maintenance of behavior change following physical activity and dietary interventions. *Health Psychology, 30,* 99–109. doi: 10.1037/a0021974

Fleig, L., Pomp, S., Schwarzer, R., & Lippke, S. (2013). Promoting exercise maintenance: How interventions with booster sessions improve long-term rehabilitation outcomes. *Rehabilitation Psychology, 58*(4), 323–333. doi: 10.1037/a0033885

Houser-Marko, L., & Sheldon, K. M. (2006). Motivating behavioral persistence: The self-as-doer construct. *Personality and Social Psychology Bulletin, 32,* 1037–1049. doi: 10.1177/0146167206287974

Jancey, J. M., Lee, A. H., Howat, P. A., Burke, L., Leong, C. C., & Shilton, T. (2011). The effectiveness of a walking booster program for seniors. *American Journal of Health Promotion, 25*(6), 363–367. doi: 10.4278/ajhp.090512-ARB-164

Metz, K., Flöter, S., Kröger, C., Donath, C., Piontek, D., & Gradl, S. (2007). Telephone booster sessions for optimizing smoking cessation for patients in rehabilitation centers. *Nicotine & Tobacco Research, 9*(8), 853–863. doi: 10.1080/14622200701485000

Miller, W. R., & Rollnick, S. (2002). *Motivational interviewing: Preparing people for change* (2nd ed.). New York: Guilford Press.

National Institutes of Health (2014). *How is heart disease treated?* Retrieved from www.nhlbi.nih.gov/health/health-topics/topics/hdw/treatment.

Prapavessis, H., Jesus, S., Fitzgeorge, L., Faulkner, G., Maddison, R., & Batten, S. (2016). Exercise to enhance smoking cessation: The getting physical on cigarette randomized control trial. *Annals of Behavioral Medicine, 50*(3), 358–369. doi: 10.1007/s12160-015-9761-9

Spohr, S. A., Nandy, R., Gandhiraj, D., Vemulapalli, A., Anne, S., & Walters, S. T. (2015). Efficacy of SMS text message interventions for smoking cessation: A meta-analysis. *Journal of Substance Abuse Treatment, 56,* 1–10. doi: 10.1016/j.jsat.2015.01.011

Stryker, S., & Burke, P. J. (2000). The past, present, and future of identity theory. *Social Psychology Quarterly, 63,* 284–297. Retrieved from www.jstor.org/stable/2695840

Appendix 6.1

Self-as-Doer Measure—Medication Behaviors

For the survey below I would like you to think about 6 goals related to taking your medication. Please write them on the first line/or in the space after each number (1, 2, 3, 4). Leave the second line/space (1b, 2b, etc.) blank until further instructions.

1. _____   1b. _____

2. _____   2b. _____

3. _____   3b. _____

4. _____   4b. _____

5. _____   5b. _____

6. _____   6b. _____

Further instructions

Every personal goal contains both a *verb* and an *object*. For example,

> For the goal "to fill my prescriptions on time" the verb is **fill** and the object is **prescriptions**.
> For the goal "to take medications at the same time every day" the verb is **take** and the object is **medications**.

I would like you to think about the verb and object in each of the goals you have and create a *special phrase* using the "-er" suffix. Place this in the second blank above (1b, 2b, 3b, etc.).

This phrase will refer to a *person who does the goal.*

> For example, the goal "to fill my prescriptions on time" might be rephrased "prescription filler."
> The goal "to take medication at the same time each day" might be rephrased "timely medication taker."

Complete this task and then read the rest of these directions (example statements can be used).

Now that you have written down your goals and the special phrase, please indicate how well the special phrase describes or fits you using the scale given below. Please put the number on the line/space in front of each number below corresponding to the above numbers.

How well does the '-er' phrase describe you?

Does Not Describe Me Well At All	Does Not Describe Me Well	Neutral	Describes Me Well	Describes Me Very Well
1	2	3	4	5

_____ 1.   _____ 3.   _____ 5.

_____ 2.   _____ 4.   _____ 6.

Index

Ajzen, I. 5
American Diabetes Association (ADA) 37–39, 59
Anderson, D. F. 46
assessment tool, self-as-doer as 74–76
attributes of self-as-doer 19–22

barriers to health behavior change 3
Beresford, S. A. 2
Brouwer, A. M. 24, 30, 37, 43–44, 48; on diabetes self-care behaviors 60, 64

chronic illness 1–2, 59–60
clinical populations 58–67; see also diabetes
creation of doer identities 29–30
Cychosz, C. 46

diabetes: development of the self-as-doer-diabetes measure for 61–64; health pilot study 60–61; self-efficacy in self-care management of 64–66; -specific self-care behaviors 36–39, 56–60
diet behaviors 1–2; change results 50–52; research on 32–34; results of the intervention impact 52–53; self-as-doer identity and 48–53

educational tool, self-as-doer as 76–78
Elliot, A. J. 28, 58
exercise identity 46–47
Exercise Identity Scale 46–47
exercise motivations 45–46
Exercise Motivations Index-2 45–46

goal creation 29

habits 23
Hastert, T. A. 2
health: consequences of poor behaviors related to 1–2; definition of 1, 8; recommendations for achieving optimal 2
health behavior change: attrition rates for 2–3; barriers to engaging in 3; in clinical populations 58–60; consequences of 2; Health Belief Model (HBM) and 3–5; importance of 42; maintenance of 83–84; Theory of Planned Behavior (TPB) and 3, 5–6; Theory of Reasoned Action (TRA) and 5–6
health behavior maintenance 83–84; difficulty of 2–3, 52
health behavior research: on diabetes-specific self-care behaviors 36–39; on diet behaviors 32–34; on physical activity behaviors 34–36
Health Belief Model (HBM) 3–5
Healthy Eating Study see diet behaviors
Houser-Marko, L. S. 18–20, 22–24, 29–30, 82

identity: exercise 46–47; self and 6–8
identity linkage 17–18
identity ratings, doer 30
identity theory 6, 16–17, 82–83
intervention, self-as-doer as 79–80

Jones, C. J. 4

Leary, M. R. 6
lifestyle modifications 2
limitations and recommendations for
   improvement of self-as-doer identity
   80–83
Llewellyn, C. 4
locus of control 23–24

maintenance, health behavior 83–84
measurement of self-as-doer identity
   29–31, 86–87
medication behaviors 86–87
Mosack, K. E. 24, 30, 48; on diabetes
   self-care behaviors 60, 64
motivation in self-as-doer identity
   44–48, 53
Muon, S. 46

National Health and Nutrition
   Examination Survey 1

outcome expectancies 24

physical activity behaviors 1;
   motivational constructs and 44–48;
   predicting 44; research on 34–36;
   self-as-doer identity and 43–48
*Physical Activity Guidelines for
   Americans* (Department of Health
   and Human Services) 43
prediction of physical activity
   behavior 44

rating of doer identities 30
Rise, J. 8
Rosenstock, I. M. 4, 7
Ruterbusch, J. J. 2

schemas 6–7
self and identity 6–8
self-as-doer-diabetes (SD-D) scale
   61–64; questions 68–70; self-efficacy
   and 64–66

self-as-doer identity 8–9; as assessment
   tool 74–76; attributes of 19–22;
   creating doer identities 29–30;
   creating goals and 29; for diabetes
   and self-efficacy in diabetes self-care
   management 64–66; diet behaviors
   and 48–53; differences between
   existing motivation and health theories
   and 22–24; as educational tool 76–78;
   examples from health behavior
   research 32–39; health behavior
   maintenance and 83–84; as identity
   linkage 17–18; as intervention 79–80;
   introduction to 16–19; limitations and
   recommendations for improvement
   of 80–83; measuring 29–31, 39–40,
   86–87; motivation and 44–48, 53;
   physical activity behaviors and
   43–48; recommendations for using
   73–84; self-efficacy and 23, 47–48;
   as self-schema 16; theoretical nature
   of 27–29; use in clinical populations
   58–67; use in various populations 74;
   versatility of 24–25
self-determination theory 22–23
self-efficacy 23, 47–48; in diabetes
   self-care management 64–66; self-
   as-doer as intervention for 79–80
self-feedback 16
Sheldon, K. 18–20, 22–24, 29–30, 82
Sheppard, L. 2
Smith, H. 4

Tangney, J. P. 6
Theory of Planned Behavior (TPB)
   3, 5–6
Theory of Reasoned Action (TRA) 5–6
triangle model of responsibility 17–18

United States Department of
   Agriculture (USDA) 49

White, E. 2
Wilson, P. M. 46
World Health Organization 1